Temporomandibular Disorders
Guidelines for Classification, Assessment, and Management

The American Academy of Orofacial Pain

Edited by
Charles McNeill, DDS

Quintessence Publishing Co, Inc
Chicago, Berlin, London, Tokyo, São Paulo, Moscow

Temporomandibular Disorders

Library of Congress Cataloging-in-Publication Data

American Academy of Orofacial Pain.
  Temporomandibular disorders : guidelines for classification,
  assessment, and management / The American Academy of
  Orofacial Pain
    edited by Charles McNeill.—2nd ed.
      p.   cm.
    Rev. ed. of: Craniomandibular Disorders. 1990.
    Includes bibliographical references.
    ISBN 0-86715-253-2
    1. Temporomandibular joint—Diseases.   I. McNeill, Charles,
  date.   II. American Academy of Craniomandibular Disorders.
  Craniomandibular Disorders.   III. Title.
  RK470.A48   1993
  617.5'22—dc20   92-37493

Second Edition

Previous edition copyrighted 1990, Craniomandibular Disorders:
Guidelines for Evaluation, Diagnosis, and Management.

Editor: Carol L. Rose
Designer and Production: Jennifer A. Sabella

Composition: Focus Graphics, St. Louis, MO
Printing and Binding: Port City Press, Baltimore, MD
Printed in the USA on recycled paper.

Contents

Preface

This document represents the recommendations of the American Academy of Orofacial Pain (AAOP), formerly known as the American Academy of Craniomandibular Disorders (AACD), for the classification, assessment, and management of temporomandibular disorders (TMD). It is a revision of the first edition of Craniomandibular Disorders: Guidelines for Evaluation, Diagnosis, and Management published by the AACD in 1990.[1] Those guidelines were an update of two prior position papers on the same subject.[2,3] The AAOP is composed of persons with academic credentials, advanced education and training, or extensive clinical experience in the field of orofacial pain and specifically in TMD.

Currently the term *temporomandibular disorders* is used interchangeably with the term *craniomandibular disorders*. However, the term temporomandibular disorders is considered the preferred term by most North American authorities in the field. The term temporomandibular disorders is specific for the orofacial region and more accurately refers to the joint and muscle problems in the area in which dentists have formal training, expertise, clinical experience, licensing, and professional and legal responsibility.[4] The term is compatible with the terminology used by the American Dental Association's TMD guidelines, numerous state dental associations' recently established TMD guidelines, and the International Headache Society's classification for headache, cranial neuralgias, and facial pain. Also, temporomandibular disorders is the term recognized by a larger percentage of the lay public and faculty and staff at multispecialty medical centers and academic institutions. Lastly, it is the term that is used by Index Medicus to classify peer-reviewed medical and dental literature.[4]

The AAOP continues to recognize an increasing need for appropriate practice guidelines, and, therefore, has published this second edition in response to the recent advances in the field. This document provides dentists, physicians, allied health professionals, researchers, and the insurance industry with a current updated review of the classification, assessment, and management of patients with TMD. The major objective is to provide guidelines based on knowledge gained from research in the basic and clinical sciences and on clinical practice experience. Literature is cited from refereed professional journals from the allied health fields in support of the guidelines. Proposed theories or clinical techniques that are not yet supported scientifically are duly noted in this publication. Because knowledge in this field is rapidly growing and changing with additional scientific research, these guidelines will continue to require periodic updating.

References

1. American Academy of Craniomandibular Disorders: McNeill C (ed) Craniomandibular disorders: Guidelines for evaluation, diagnosis, and management. J Craniomandib Disord Oral Facial Pain. Chicago, Quintessence Publishing Co, 1990.

2. McNeill C, Danzig WM, Farrar WB, Gelb H, Lerman M, Moffett BC, Pertes R, Solberg WK, Weinberg L: Craniomandibular (TMJ) disorders—The state of the art. J Prosthet Dent 1980;44:434–437.

3. McNeill C: Craniomandibular (TMJ) disorders—The state of the art, Part II: Accepted diagnosis and treatment modalities. J Prosthet Dent 1983;49:393–397.

4. McNeill C (ed): Current Controversies in Temporomandibular Disorders. Chicago, Quintessence Publishing Co, 1992.

AAOP "Guidelines" Committee Members
1990–1992

Charles McNeill, DDS, Chairman

James R. Fricton, DDS, MS
Joseph A. Gibilisco, DDS, MSD
Steven B. Graff-Radford, DDS
Tore L. Hansson, DDS, Odont Dr
James A. Howard, DDS

Eric K. Milliner, MD
Jeffrey P. Okeson, DMD
Harold T. Perry, DDS, PhD
John D. Rugh, PhD
Donald A. Seligman, DDS

ONE

Introduction

Definition of TMD

Temporomandibular disorders (TMD) is a collective term embracing a number of clinical problems that involve the masticatory musculature, the temporomandibular joint (TMJ) and associated structures, or both. The term is synonymous with the term *craniomandibular disorders*. Temporomandibular disorders have been identified as a major cause of nondental pain in the orofacial region and are considered to be a subclassification of musculoskeletal disorders.[1] Although TMD was viewed as one syndrome, current research supports the view that TMD are a cluster of related disorders in the masticatory system that have many common symptoms.[2,3]

The most frequent presenting symptom is pain, usually localized in the muscles of mastication, the preauricular area, and/or the TMJ. The pain usually is aggravated by chewing or other jaw function. In addition to complaints of pain, patients with these disorders frequently have limited or asymmetric mandibular movement and TMJ sounds that are most frequently described as clicking, popping, grating, or crepitus.

Common patient complaints include jaw ache, earache, headache, and facial pain. Nonpainful masticatory muscle hypertrophy and abnormal occlusal wear associated with oral parafunction such as *bruxism* (jaw clenching and tooth grinding) may be related problems. Pain or dysfunction due to nonmusculoskeletal causes such as otolaryngologic, neurologic, vascular, neoplastic, or infectious disease in the orofacial region is not considered a primary temporomandibular disorder even though musculoskeletal pain may be present. However, TMD often coexist with other craniofacial and orofacial pain disorders.

History of TMD

A historical review of TMD reveals a notable evolutionary process given considerable impetus following the publication in

1934 of a paper by Costen, an otolaryngologist.[4] Costen observed that patients with pain in or near the ear, tinnitus, dizziness, a sensation of ear pressure or fullness, and difficulty in swallowing (known as *Costen's Syndrome*) seemed to improve by altering the vertical dimension of the occlusion. Because malocclusion was perceived to be the underlying cause, treatment for TMD and a variety of other orofacial pain phenomenon shifted from medicine to dentistry. Dental occlusionists contended shortly thereafter that occlusal disharmony rather than a closed bite was the primary etiologic factor,[5] and various restorative techniques to balance or stabilize the occlusion resulted during the period from the late 1930s to the post–World War II era.

Studies were expanding in the fields of neuromuscular physiology[6,7] and joint biomechanics including dysfunction, remodeling, and degenerative processes.[8–10] Other clinical investigators were emphasizing different approaches to the management of head, neck, and orofacial pain and TMD. Regional and referred pain of myofascial origin was considered to be a major influence in these conditions.[11–13] Conversely, the gnathologic approach, as described by McCollum and Stuart,[14] emphasized the importance of occlusion and the TMJs.

The role of occlusion in TMD gained in popularity from the late 1950s with an emphasis on occlusal equilibration or adjustment.[15–17] In the 1960s the quality of clinical investigation and basic scientific research was becoming increasingly sophisticated[18–20] and there was a gradual de-emphasis of the role of occlusion in TMD etiology.

After 1970, advances in imaging techniques that included tomography, arthrography,[21,22] computed tomography (CT),[23] and, later, magnetic resonance imaging (MRI),[24–27] resulted in improved visualization of intracapsular structures. Farrar[28] challenged the neuromuscular oriented concepts and reemphasized the joint condition, especially disc interference disorders, as demonstrated by arthrography and supported by the surgical findings of McCarty.[29] Wilkes[30] also described articular disorders stating the importance of arthrographic soft tissue imaging and surgery. These imaging techniques, especially MRI, and arthroscopy[31–34] plus increasing experience in clinical management, provided information for more specific articular diagnoses.

At this time multidisciplinary knowledge was leading to more refined differential diagnoses and the realization that orofacial pain patients may suffer from a variety of disorders including systemic-related problems and articular, neuromuscular, neurologic, neurovascular, and behavioral disorders. Parallel to the development of knowledge in TMD, there has been an expansion of knowledge in the basic mechanisms of pain and major advances in the neurophysiology and neuropharmacology of pain.

It became evident that diagnostic and management guidelines were of paramount importance in the 1980s, a decade characterized by a proliferation of TMD devices, both diagnostic and therapeutic. Accordingly, in 1982 the American Dental Association (ADA) held a conference on the examination, diagnosis, and management of TMD.[3] The need for an improved classification system that would permit proper comparison of epidemiologic, diagnostic, and treatment data was stressed. It was also recognized that some patients developed a lingering, chronic, painful illness with an unpredictable treatment response to modalities usually found effective in managing biomechanical, structural dysfunctions. The complexity of managing a chronic orofacial pain disorder was acknowledged and the use of multidisciplinary and interdisciplinary management programs became common.

Anatomy of the Masticatory System

Craniomandibular articulation occurs in the temporomandibular joints, two of the most complex joints of the body. Each TMJ provides for hinging movement in one plane, which is a criterion for a *ginglymoid joint*. At the same time, however, the TMJ provides for gliding movements, which is a criterion for an *arthrodial joint*. Thus, the TMJ is technically considered a *ginglymoarthrodial joint*.[2] The TMJ is formed by the mandibular condyle fitting into the mandibular fossa of the temporal

bone (Fig 1-1). Separating these two bones from direct contact is the interposed articular disc (sometimes inappropriately referred to as "meniscus"). The healthy articular portion of the disc is composed of dense fibrous connective tissue, devoid of any nerves or vessels; conversely, the posterior attachment of the disc is richly vascularized and innervated.[35–37] The disc is also attached to the condyle both medially and laterally by collateral ligaments. These ligaments permit rotational movement of the disc on the condyle during opening and closing of the mouth. This so-called condyle-disc complex translates out of the fossa during extended mouth opening (Fig 1-2).[2] Therefore, in the normal joint, rotational movement occurs between the condyle and the infe-

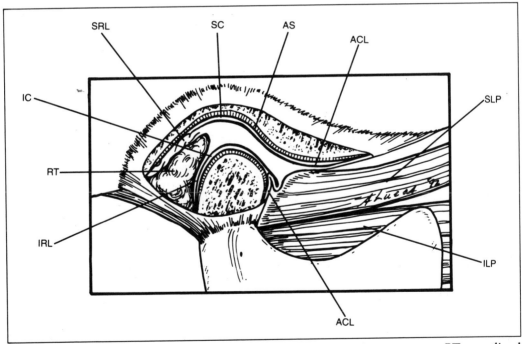

Fig 1-1 Temporomandibular joint. Diagram showing the anatomic components: *RT*, retrodiscal tissues; *SRL*, superior retrodiscal lamina (elastic); *IRL*, inferior retrodiscal lamina (collagenous); *ACL*, anterior capsular ligament (collagenous); *SLP* and *ILP*, superior and inferior lateral pterygoid muscles; *AS*, articular surface; *SC* and *IC*, superior and inferior joint cavity; *DL*, discal (collateral) ligament. Figure reproduced with permission from Okeson JP: Management of Temporomandibular Disorders and Occlusion, ed 3. St Louis, CV Mosby Co, 1992, fig 1-14.

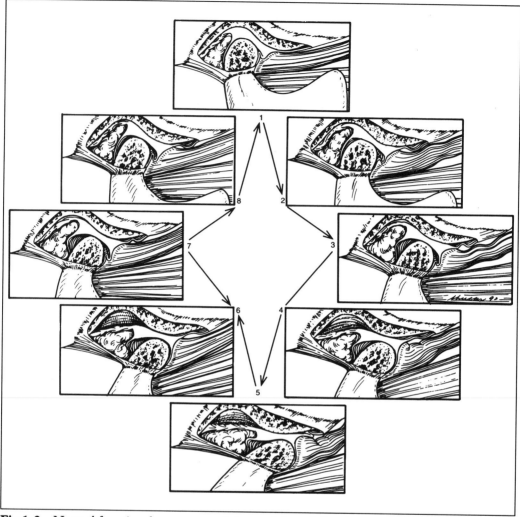

Fig 1-2 Normal functional movement of the condyle and disc during the full range of opening and closing. Note that the disc is rotated posteriorly on the condyle as the condyle is translated out of the fossa. The closing movement is the exact opposite of opening. Figure reproduced with permission from Okeson JP: Management of Temporomandibular Disorders and Occlusion, ed 3. St Louis, CV Mosby Co, 1992, fig 1-27.

rior surface of the disc during early opening (the inferior joint space) and translation takes place in the space between the superior surface of the disc and the fossa (the superior joint space) during later opening. Movement of the joint is lubricated by synovial fluid, which also acts as a medium for transporting nutrients to and waste products from the articular surfaces.

Unlike most synovial joints, the articulator surfaces of the TMJs are lined with dense fibrous connective tissue, not hyaline cartilage.[38] This is an important feature because fibrous connective tissue has a greater ability to repair itself than does hyaline cartilage. This implies that the management of arthritic conditions of the TMJ may be dif-

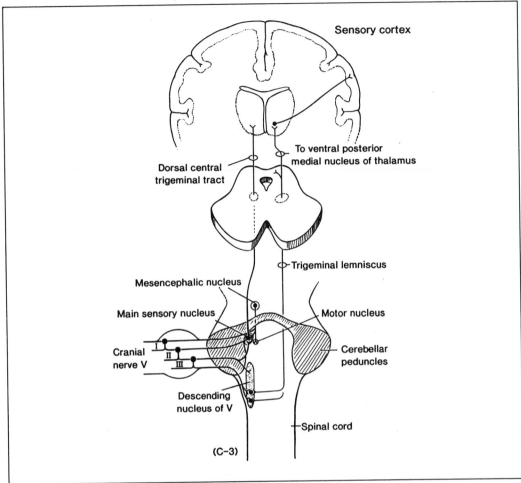

Fig 1-3 Central trigeminal sensory pathways. Dorsal view of spinal, brain stem, thalamic, and cortical pain temperature/touch pathways. The ascending trigeminal tract (lemniscus) is the primary pain/temperature pathway while the dorsal central trigeminal tract conveys most of the touch impulses.

ferent from that of other synovial joints.[39]

Movement and stability of the TMJs is achieved by a group of skeletal muscles referred to as the muscles of mastication. Although the muscles of mastication are the primary muscles that provide mandibular movement, other associated muscles of the head and neck furnish secondary support during mastication. The masticatory muscles include the *masseter*, *medial pterygoid*, and *temporal muscles*, which predominantly elevate the mandible (mouth closing); the *digastric muscles*, which assist in mandibular depression (mouth opening); the *inferior lateral pterygoid muscles*, which assist in protruding the mandible; and the *superior lateral pterygoid muscles*, which provide stabilization for the condyle and disc during function.[40–42] The masticatory muscles are recruited in a variety of functional behaviors that includes talking, swallowing, and masticating.[43] A number of muscle behaviors are also apparently nonfunctional (parafunctional), defined under the broad term of bruxism, and include grinding, clenching, or rhythmic chewing-like, empty-mouth movements.[44,45]

Motor innervation of the muscles of mastication as well as sensory innervation to the oral structures and the face are supplied by the trigeminal cranial nerve (CV). Sensory fibers of the trigeminal nerve extend to synapses in the trigeminal spinal nucleus of the brain stem. It is important to appreciate that the anatomy of this spinal nucleus extends caudally down into the region where cervical nerves 1 through 3 enter the central nervous system. Neurons from the trigeminal as well as facial (CVII), hypoglossal (CIX), and vagus (CX) cranial nerves share in the same neuron pool as neurons from the upper cervical spine (cervical nerves 1, 2, 3) (Fig 1-3).[46–49] This convergence of the trigeminal and cervical nerves is an anatomic and physiologic explanation for the source of referred pain from the cervical region to the trigeminal region.[50] The clinician needs to be aware of this common referral pattern so as to avoid misdirected diagnosis and treatment.

References

1. Bell WE: Orofacial pains. Classification, Diagnosis, Management. 4th ed. Chicago, Year Book Medical Publishers, 1989, pp 101–113.

2. Bell WE: Temporomandibular Disorders. Classification, Diagnosis, Management. 3rd ed. Chicago, Year Book Medical Publishers, 1990, pp 166–176.

3. Griffiths RH: Report of the President's Conference on Examination, Diagnosis and Management of Temporomandibular Disorders. J Am Dent Assoc 1983;106:75–77.

4. Costen JB: A syndrome of ear and sinus symptoms dependent upon disturbed function of the temporomandibular joint. Ann Otol 1934;43:1–15.

5. Schuyler CH: Fundamental principles in the correction of occlusal disharmony, natural and artificial. J Am Dent Assoc 1935;22:1193–1202.

6. Moyers RE: An electromyographic analysis of certain muscles involved in temporomandibular movement. Am J Orthod 1950;36:481–515.

7. Perry HT: Implications of myographic research. Angle Orthod 1955;25:179.

8. Moffett BC, Johnson LC, McCabe JB, et al: Articular remodeling in the adult human temporomandibular joint. Am J Anat 1964;115:119–130.

9. Blackwood HJJ: Cellular remodeling in articular tissue. J Dent Res 1966;45:480–489.

10. Carlsson GE, Oberg T: Remodeling of the temporomandibular joint. Oral Sci Rev 1974;4:53–86.

11. Travell J, Rinzler SH: The myofascial genesis of pain. Postgrad Med 1952;11:425–434.

12. Schwartz LL: Pain associated with the temporomandibular joint. J Am Dent Assoc 1955;51:394–397.

13. Laskin DM: Etiology of the pain-dysfunction syndrome. J Am Dent Assoc 1969;79:147–153.

14. McCollum BB, Stuart CE: A research report. South Pasadena, Calif, Scientific Press, 1955.

15. Shore NA: Occlusal Equilibration and Temporomandibular Joint Dysfunction. Philadelphia, JB Lippincott Co, 1959, pp 201–270.

16. Ramfjord SP: Dysfunctional temporomandibular joint and muscle pain. J Prosthet Dent 1961;11:353–374.

17. Krough-Poulson WG, Olsson A: Occlusal disharmonies and dysfunction of the stomatognathic system. Dent Clin North Am Nov 1966;627–635.

18. Thilander B: Innervation of the temporomandibular joint capsule in man. Trans

Royal School Dent (Stockholm and Umea) 1961;7:9–67.

19. Kawamura Y, Majima T: Temporomandibular joint's sensory mechanisms controlling activities of the jaw muscles. J Dent Res 1964;43:150.

20. Storey AT: Sensory functions of the temporomandibular joint. Can Dent Assoc J 1968;34:294–300.

21. Dolwick MR, Katzberg RW, Helms CA, Bales DJ: Arthrotomographic evaluation of the temporomandibular joint. J Oral Maxillofac Surg 1979;37:793–799.

22. Katzberg RW, Dolwick MF, Helms CA, Hopens T, Bales DJ, Coggs GC: Arthrotomography of the temporomandibular joint. AJR 1980;134:995–1003.

23. Helms CA, Katzberg RW, Manzione JV: Computed tomography. In Helms CA, Katzberg RW, Dolwick MF (eds) Internal Derangements of the Temporomandibular Joint. San Francisco, Radiology Research Foundation, 1983, pp 135–166.

24. Helms CA, Morrish RB, Kircos LT, Katzberg RW, Dolwick WF: Computed tomography of the meniscus temporomandibular joint: Preliminary observations. Radiology 1982;145:719–722.

25. Harms SE, Wilk RM, Wolfford LM, Chiles DG, Milan SB: The temporomandibular joint: Magnetic resonance imaging using surface coils. Radiology 1985;157:133–136.

26. Helms CA, Kaban LB, McNeill C, Dobson T: Temporomandibular joint: Morphology and signal intensity characteristics of the disc at MR imaging. Radiology 1989; 172:817–820.

27. Helms CA, Doyle GW, Orwig D, McNeill C, Kaban L: Staging of internal derangements of the TMJ with magnetic resonance imaging: Preliminary observations. J Craniomandib Disord Facial Oral Pain 1989;3: 93–99.

28. Farrar WB: Diagnosis and treatment of anterior dislocation of the articular disc. NY J Dent 1971;41:348–351.

29. McCarty W: Diagnosis and treatment of internal derangements of the articular disc

and mandibular condyle. In Solberg WK, Clark GT (eds) Temporomandibular Joint Problems: Biologic Diagnosis and Treatment. Chicago, Quintessence Publ Co, 1980, pp 145–168.

30. Wilkes CH: Arthrography of the temporomandibular joint. Minn Med 1978;61:645–652.

31. Kino K: Morphological and structural observations of the synovial membranes and their folds relating to the endoscope findings in the upper joint cavity of the human temporomandibular joint (in Japanese). J Stomatol Soc Jpn 1980;47:98–134.

32. Ohnishi M: Clinical applications of the arthroscope in temporomandibular joint diseases. Bull Tokyo Med/Dent Univ 1980, pp 141–150.

33. Murakami K-I, Matsuki M, Iizuka T, Ono T: Diagnostic arthroscopy of the TMJ: Differential diagnosis in patients with limited jaw opening. J Craniomand Pract 1986; 4:118–126.

34. Sanders B: Arthroscopic surgery of the temporomandibular joint: Treatment of internal derangement with persistent closed lock. Oral Surg Oral Med Oral Pathol 1986; 62:361–372.

35. Fried L: Anatomy of the Head, Neck, Face and Jaws. Lea and Febiger, Philadelphia, 1980, pp 43–83; 173–186.

36. Scapino RP: The posterior attachment: Its structure, function, and appearance in TMJ imaging studies. Part I. J Craniomandib Disord Facial Oral Pain 1991;5:83–95.

37. Scapino RP: The posterior attachment: Its structure, function, and appearance in TMJ imaging studies. Part 2. J Craniomandib Disord Facial Oral Pain 1991;5:155–166.

38. Dubrul E: The craniomandibular articulation. In Sicher's Oral Anatomy. 7th ed. St Louis, CV Mosby Co, 1980, Chap 4, pp 147–209.

39. Meikle MC: Remodeling. In Sarnat BG, Laskin DM (ed) The Temporomandibular Joint: A Biological Basis for Clinical Practice. 4th ed. WB Saunders Co, Philadelphia, 1992, pp 93–107.

40. McNamara JA: The independent functions of the two heads of the lateral pterygoid muscles. Am J Anat 1973;138:197–206.

41. Meyenberg K, Kubik S, Palla S: Relationships of the muscles of mastication to the articular disc of the temporomandibular joint. Helv Odont Acta 1986;30:1–20.

42. Wilkinson TM: The relationship between the disk and the lateral pterygoid muscle in the human temporomandibular joint. J Prosthet Dent 1988;60:715–724.

43. Hylander WL: Functional anatomy. In Saranat BG and Laskin DM (eds), The Temporomandibular Joint: A Biological Basis for Clinical Practice. 4th ed. Philadelphia, WB Saunders Co, 1992, pp 60–92.

44. Glaros AG, Rao SM: Effects of bruxism: A review of the literature. J Prosthet Dent 1977;38:149–157.

45. Rugh JD, Harlan J: Nocturnal bruxism and temporomandibular disorders. Adv Neurol 1988;49:329–341.

46. Kerr FWL: Structural relation of the trigeminal spinal tract to upper cervical roots and the solitary nucleus in the cat. Exp Neurol 1961;4:134.

47. Kerr FWL: Facial, vagal and glossopharyngeal nerves in the cat: Afferent connections. Arch Neurol 1962;6:264.

48. Kerr FWL: The divisional organization of afferent fibers of the trigeminal nerve. Brain 1963;86:721.

49. Sessle BJ: The neurobiology of facial and dental pain: Present knowledge, future directions. J Dent Res 1987;66:962–981.

50. Giunta JL, Kronman JH: Orofacial involvement secondary to trapezius muscle trauma. Oral Surg Oral Med Oral Pathol 1985; 60:368–369.

Epidemiology

Epidemiology is the study of the factors that govern the frequency and distribution of disease or physiologic states in a community.[1] Its focus is on the total population rather than the individual,[2] and its purpose is disease classification and prevention.[3] Epidemiologic studies can be descriptive or analytic. Descriptive investigation usually involves retrospective evaluation of the number of cases with any disease or associated factor. These findings are reported as *prevalence*. Analytic investigation usually involves prospective longitudinal evaluation of the number of cases acquiring a disease or an associated factor over a specified time period. These findings are reported as *incidence*. Few reports on the incidence of TMD and the associated signs and symptoms are available, so the emphasis in this chapter will be, by default, on prevalence. However, the majority of studied populations are cross-sectional samples and are not necessarily representative of broader populations. Thus, few are strict epidemiologic studies of total populations and the findings, therefore, cannot easily be generalized to more global communities.

TMD

Cross-sectional epidemiologic studies of specific nonpatient populations show that approximately 75% of those populations have at least one sign of joint dysfunction (movement abnormalities, joint noise, tenderness on palpation, etc) and approximately 33% have at least one symptom (face pain, joint pain, etc).[4,5] The results from epidemiologic studies vary considerably from study to study because of differences in descriptive terminology, in data collection, in analytic approaches (eg, single-factor versus multiple-factor analysis), and in the individual factors selected for study.

Some signs appear to be relatively common in healthy populations: joint sounds or deviation on mouth opening occur in approximately 50% of healthy nonpatient populations. Other signs are relatively rare: mouth opening limitations only occur in approximately 5%.[6] Signs and symptoms of TMD generally increase in frequency and severity beginning in the second decade of life.[7–9] The incidence of joint sounds in young adults in their late teens can be as high as 17.5% over a 2-year period.[10] The majority of 3,428 patients in a recent study were between the ages of 15 and 45 years (mean, 32.9 years); this suggests that older subjects are less bothered by their symptoms.[11]

Prevalence of nonspecific measures of overall symptom levels (eg, Helkimo indices) was reported to be almost equal in men and women in Scandinavian nonpatient surveys of adults[12–16] and younger populations.[17–21] In contrast, when individual symptoms were evaluated separately, women were found to have slightly more headache, TMJ clicking, TMJ tenderness, and muscle tenderness than were men.[8,9,22–24] These differences between men and women found in epidemiologic studies only partially explain the recent clinical tabulations stating a women-to-men ratio of 3:1 to 9:1 in persons seeking care for TMD.[11,25,26] Temporomandibular disorders are often remitting, self-limiting, or fluctuating over time as suggested by recent patient studies.[27,28] While knowledge of the natural history or course of TMD is limited, there is increasing evidence that progression to chronic and disabling intracapsular TMJ disease is an uncommon occurrence.[29]

Despite the large percentages of the population having signs or symptoms (see Fig 2-1), only 5% to 7% are estimated to be in need of treatment.[3,4,30–32] These estimates are supported by a recent study that indicated that only 7% of a patient population with nonproblematic TMJ clicking showed progression to a problematic clicking status over a 1- to 7.5-year period.[28] The majority of the patients with TMJ clicking remained stable or showed less or no clicking over the examination period even though most did not have any treatment interventions. Furthermore, while TMJ clicking is fairly common, the progression to a potentially more serious nonreducing disc status is relatively uncommon.[27] It is unfortunate that the incidence of disc displacement without reduction is not currently known and, further, that the progression from locking to osteoarthrosis or significant disability is variable. Because MRI has made documentation of disc derangement without invasive procedures available, the question of disability potential is clinically important to avoid overtreatment of benign chronic nonreducing disc displacement. The internal derangement–osteoarthrosis-disability continuum is thus less predictable and more complex than was previously proposed by Rasmussen.[33,34]

The prevalence of a specific temporomandibular disorder is difficult to determine because of the lack of a universally accepted classification scheme with diagnostic criteria. However, different investigators have used combinations of signs and symptoms to indirectly deduce the prevalence of differentiated diagnoses. A recent study of patients seeking treatment for TMD in a private dental practice described 31% with internal derangement, 39% with arthritis, and 30% with a muscle disorder.[35] Schiffman et al[30] used specifically tested diagnostic criteria on a general population and found 33% with TMD and 41% with masticatory muscle disorders but only 7% of the total population had a disorder severe enough to be comparable to a clinic population. Thus, prevalence values of patients may overstate the clinical significance of individual problems because patients with mild transient signs and symptoms not requiring treatment are no doubt included.

To overcome the shortcomings of past

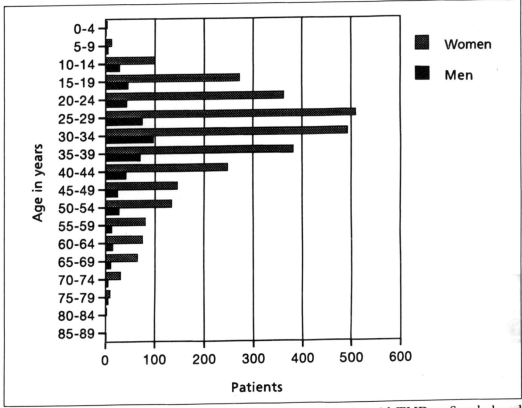

Fig 2-1 Age and sex distribution of 3,428 TMD patients presenting with TMD at a Seattle-based health maintenance organization of 360,000 enrollees. The mean ages of the women and men were 34.2 years and 33.8 years, respectively, and, of those seeking treatment, 85.4% were women. (Figure adapted with permission, originally appeared as Fig 4.1 in Howard.[11])

studies of prevalence, a universally accepted classification scheme with case definitions such as is proposed in these guidelines is mandatory.[36] In addition, the development of an impairment-disability scale is recommended to allow comparative cross-study estimates. Finally, while broad-based symptom scales (eg, the Helkimo indices) have been useful in the past, recent advances in disorder classification mandate that future epidemiologic studies, using working definitions that include patterns of signs and symptoms, focus on more narrowly defined disease groups.

Chronic Pain Disorders

Although most TMD appear to be mild and self-limiting, a significant number of TMD patients develop a *chronic pain syndrome*.[36] Chronic pain syndromes are defined as persistent pain that lasts more than 6 months with associated behavioral and psychosocial factors.[37,38] There is increasing recognition of the need for epidemiologic studies of the prevalence and impact of chronic and recurrent pain.[39]

One comprehensive survey examining chronic pain prevalence among adults in North America suggests that there is value in comparing different pain conditions.[40,41] In this study, various pain conditions were found to share common features such as age distribution and association with psychologic stress. The findings also indicate that having had a pain condition in the preceding 12 months is common in the adult North American population, with 73% experiencing headache, 56% experiencing back pain, 46% experiencing stomach pain, and 27% experiencing dental pain. Another study on the prevalence of pain found that by 70 years of age, 34% have experienced significant headache, abdominal pain, or chest pain.[42] Headaches, facial pain, and most other chronic pains are more prevalent among women.[8,9,24]

Chronic pain involves long-term nociceptive input with complex central and peripheral nervous system changes at levels of both perception and reaction.[43] Patient response to chronic pain is different from acute pain response.[44] Ongoing peripheral pathology is potentiated by neuropsychologic factors, such as social situations, attitudes, and emotional problems, and may cause an enhanced perception of continuous pain. Some patients with chronic pain are able to cope with this continuous unpleasant perception and manage to live productive lives.[45] When their coping mechanisms break down, however, patients may become depressed, disabled, and dependent on the pain regardless of the original event that started the pain problem. These patients have complex pain and are often victims of multiple unsuccessful treatments, which include multiple drug misuse and surgical interventions for pain.[46]

Headache

Headache can be a symptom of many disorders affecting the masticatory system. Many studies have found recurrent headache to occur in as many as 70% of TMD patients,[47,48] compared to approximately 20% of a general population.[49–51] It has been estimated that one in three persons suffers from severe headache at some stage in his or her life.[52] Currently, 5% to 10% of the North American population has sought medical advice for severe headache.[41,53] There is also a high prevalence in children; 75% of Scandinavian children report histories of significant head pain by age 15.[54]

Because headache is a major cause of suffering and absenteeism from work or school,[40,41] epidemiologic studies of headache are needed to clarify the relationship with TMD. Temporomandibular disorders do not necessarily cause headache and there is need for study of the possibility that TMD aggravates headache in those patients predisposed to headache. An association between the presence of headache and TMD has been well documented,[47,49,55–60] but this association has not yet shown to be a causal relationship and may be coincidental in many cases. Clarification of the role of the musculoskeletal system in producing headache is not currently available. Thus, it is important to emphasize that headache per se should not be considered a temporomandibular disorder unless the pain is clearly related to clinical signs and symptoms that involve the masticatory musculoskeletal system.

References

1. Arey LB, Burrows W, Greenhill JP, Hewitt RM (eds): Dorland's Illustrated Medical Dictionary. 23rd ed. Philadelphia, WB Saunders Co, 1960.

2. Zwemer TJ (ed): Boucher's Clinical Dental Terminology. St Louis, CV Mosby Co, 1982.

3. Solberg WK: Epidemiology, Incidence, and Prevalence of Temporomandibular Disorders: A Review. The President's Conference on the Examination, Diagnosis, and Management of Temporomandibular Disorders. Chicago, American Dental Association, 1983, pp 30–39.

4. Rugh JD, Solberg WK: Oral health status in the United States. Temporomandibular disorders. J Dent Educ 1985;49:398–404.

5. Schiffman E, Fricton JR: Epidemiology of TMJ and craniofacial pain. In Friction JR, Kroening RJ, Hathaway KM (eds) TMJ and Craniofacial Pain: Diagnosis and Management. St Louis, IEA Publ, 1988, pp 1–10.

6. Huber MA, Hall EH: A comparison of the signs of temporomandibular joint dysfunction and occlusal discrepancies in a symptom-free population of men and women. Oral Surg Oral Med Oral Pathol 1990;70:180–183.

7. Egermark-Eriksson I, Carlsson GE, Magnusson T: A long-term epidemiologic study of the relationship between occlusal factors and mandibular dysfunction in children and adolescents. J Dent Res 1987;67:67–71.

8. Agerberg G, Bergenholz A: Craniomandibular disorders in adult populations of West Bothnia, Sweden. Acta Odontol Scand 1989;47:129–140.

9. Salonen L, Hellden L: Prevalence of signs and symptoms of dysfunction in the masticatory system: An epidemiologic study in an adult Swedish population. J Craniomandib Disord Facial Oral Pain 1990;4:241–250.

10. Wänman A, Agerberg G: Temporomandibular joint sounds in adolescents, a longitudinal study. Oral Surg Oral Med Oral Pathol 1990;69:2–9.

11. Howard JA: Temporomandibular joint disorders, facial pain and dental problems of performing artists. In Sataloff R, Brandfonbrener A, Lederman R (eds) Textbook of Performing Arts Medicine. New York, Raven Press, 1991, pp 111–169.

12. Agerberg G, Carlsson GE: Functional disorders of the masticatory system. I. Distribution of symptoms according to age and sex as judged from investigation by questionnaire. Acta Odontol Scand 1972;30:597–613.

13. Helkimo M: Studies on function and dysfunction of the masticatory system. I: An epidemiological investigation of symptoms of dysfunction in Lapps in the North of Finland. Proc Finn Dent Soc 1974;70:37–49.

14. Helkimo M: Studies of function and dysfunction of the masticatory system. II: Index for anamnestic and clinical dysfunction and occlusal state. Swed Dent J 1974;67:101–121.

15. Hansson T, Nilner M: A study of the occurrence of symptoms of diseases of the temporomandibular joint, masticatory musculature, and related structures. J Oral Rehabil 1975;2:313–324.

16. Swanljung O, Rantanen T: Functional disorders of the masticatory system in southwest Finland. Community Dent Oral Epidemiol 1979;7(3):177–182.

17. Egermark-Eriksson I, Carlsson GE, Ingervall B: Prevalence of mandibular dysfunction and orofacial parafunction in 7-, 11-, and 15-year old Swedish children. Eur J Orthod 1981;3(3):163–172.

18. Nilner M, Lassing SA: Prevalence of functional disturbances and diseases of the stomatognathic system in 7–14 year olds. Swed Dent J 1981;5:173–187.

19. Nilner M: Prevalence of functional disturbances and diseases of the stomatognathic system in 15–18 year olds. Swed Dent J 1981;5:189–197.

20. Heft MW: Prevalence of TMJ signs and symptoms in the elderly. Gerontology 1984;3:125–130.

21. Magnusson T, Egermark-Eriksson I, Carlsson G: Five year longitudinal study of signs and symptoms of mandibular dysfunction in adolescents. J Craniomand Pract 1986;4:339–343.

22. Solberg WK, Woo MW, Houston JB: Prevalence of mandibular dysfunction in young adults. J Am Dent Assoc 1979;98:25–34.

23. Pullinger A, Seligman DA, Solberg W: Temporomandibular disorders. Part I: Functional status, dentomorphologic features, and sex differences in a nonpatient population. J Prosthet Dent 1988;59:228–235.

24. Agerberg G, Inkapööl I: Craniomandibular disorders in an urban Swedish population. J Craniomandib Disord Facial Oral Pain 1990;4:154–164.

25. McNeill C: The optimum temporomandibular joint condyle position in clinical practice. Int J Periodont Rest Dent 1985; 5(6):53–76.

26. Centore L, Bianchi P, McNeill C: The relationship between nonorganic multiple physical complaints and narcissism. J Dent Res 1989;68(special issue):abstr 317.

27. Pullinger A, Seligman D: TMJ osteoarthrosis: A differentiation of diagnostic subgroups by symptom history and demographics. J Craniomandib Disord Facial Oral Pain 1987;1:251–256.

28. Randolph CS, Greene CS, Moretti R, Forbes D, Perry HT: Conservative management of temporomandibular disorders: A post treatment comparison between patients from a university clinic and from private practice. Am J Orthod Dentofac Orthop 1990;98:77–82.

29. Nickerson JW, Boering G: Natural course of osteoarthrosis as it relates to internal derangement of the temporomandibular joint. Oral Maxillofac Surg Clin North Am 1989;1:1–19.

30. Schiffman E, Fricton JR, Haley D, Shapiro BL: The prevalence and treatment needs of subjects with temporomandibular disorders. J Am Dent Assoc 1989;120:295–304.

31. Dworkin SF, LeResche LR, Von Korff, Howard J, Truelove E, Sommers E: Epidemiology of signs and symptoms in temporomandibular disorders: I. Clinical signs in cases and controls. J Am Dent Assoc 1990;120:273–281.

32. Greene CS, Marbach JJ: Epidemiologic studies of mandibular dysfunction: A critical review. J Prosthet Dent 1982;48(2):184–190.

33. Rasmussen CO: Clinical findings during the course of temporomandibular arthropathy. Scand J Dent Res 1981;89:283–288.

34. Nitzan DW, Dolwick MF: An alternative explanation for the genesis of closed-lock symptoms in the internal derangement process. J Oral Maxillofac Surg 1991;49:810–815.

35. Pullinger A, Seligman DA: Overbite and overjet characteristics of refined diagnostic groups of temporomandibular patients. Am J Orthod Dentofac Orthop 1991;100:401–415.

36. LeResche L, Dworkin SF, Sommers EE, Truelove EL: An epidemiologic evaluation of two diagnostic classification schemes for temporomandibular disorders. J Prosthet Dent 1991;65:131–137.

37. Sanders SH: Chronic pain: Conceptualization and epidemiology. Ann Behav Med 1985;7:3–5.

38. Merskey H: Classification of chronic pain—descriptions of chronic pain syndromes and definitions of pain terms. Pain 1986;(suppl 3):1–225.

39. National Institute of Health Consensus Development Conference. The Integrated Approach to the Management of Pain. NIH Consensus Development Conference Statement. Vol 6 No. 3, Washington, DC, US Government Printing Office, 1986.

40. Sternbach RA: Pain and "hassles" in the United States: Findings of the Nuprin pain report. Pain 1986;27:69–80.

41. Sternbach RA: Survey of pain in the United States: The Nuprin Pain Report. Clin J Pain 1986;2:49–53.

42. Dworkin SF, Burgess JA: Orofacial pain of psychogenic origin: Current concepts and classification. J Am Dent Assoc 1987;115:565–571.

43. Fields HL: Pain. New York, McGraw Hill Book Co, 1987, pp 145–158.

44. Hagberg C, Hellsing G, Hagberg M: Perception of cutaneous electrical stimulation in patients with craniomandibular disorders. J Craniomandib Disord Facial Oral Pain 1990;4:120–125.

45. Turk DC, Rudy TE: Towards a comprehensive assessment of chronic pain patients. Behav Res Ther 1987;25:237–249.

46. Brena SF, Chapman SL: Management of Patients with Chronic Pain. New York, SP Medical and Scientific Books (a division of Spectrum Publications, Inc), 1982, pp 25–27.

47. Magnusson T, Carlsson GE: Comparison between two groups of patients in respect to headache and mandibular dysfunction. Swed Dent J 1978;2:85–87.

48. Andrasik F, Holyroyd KA, Abell T: Prevalence of headache within a college student population: A preliminary analysis. Headache 1979;19:384–387.

49. Magnusson T, Carlsson GE: Recurrent headaches in relation to temporomandibular joint pain-dysfunction. Acta Odontol Scand 1978;36:333–338.

50. Rieder C: The incidence of some occlusal habits and headaches/neckaches in an initial survey population. J Prosthet Dent 1976;35:445–451.

51. Turner D, Stone A: Headache and its treatment: A random sample survey. Headache 1979;19:74–77.

52. National Institute of Health Ad Hoc Committee on Classification of Headache. JAMA 1962;179:717–718.

53. Campbell JK: Headache in adults: An overview. J Craniomandib Disord Facial Oral Pain 1987;1:11–15.

54. Bille, B: Migraine in school children. Acta Pediatr 1962;51:13–147.

55. Helöe B, and Helöe LA: Frequency and distribution of myofascial pain-dysfunction syndrome in a population of 25-year-olds. Community Dent Oral Epidemiol 1979; 7:357–360.

56. Isberg A, Widmalm S-E, Ivarsson R: Clinical, radiographic, and electromyographic study of patients with internal derangement of the temporomandibular joint. Am J Orthod 1985;88:453–460.

57. Wänman A, Agerberg G: Headache and dysfunction of the masticatory system in adolescents. Cephalgia 1986;6:247–255.

58. Förssell H: Mandibular dysfunction and headache. Thesis. Turku, Finland, University of Turku. Finn Dent Soc 1985;81 (suppl 2).

59. Schokker RP, Hansson TL, Ansink BJJ: Craniomandibular disorders in patients with different types of headache. J Craniomandib Disord Facial Oral Pain 1990;4:47–51.

60. Schokker RP, Hansson TL, Ansink BJJ: The result of treatment of the masticatory system of chronic headache patients. J Craniomandib Disord Facial Oral Pain 1990; 4:126–130.

THREE

Etiology

Most of the etiologic factors discussed in this chapter can be considered to have merely an association with TMD. These contributing factors thought to be clinically relevant await future research to document their etiologic significance. Because TMD are diverse and often multifactorial, a universal etiology of TMD does not exist.

Factors that increase the risk of TMD are called *predisposing*. Factors that cause the onset of TMD are called *initiating*. Factors that interfere with healing or enhance the progression of TMD are called *perpetuating*. Individual factors, under different circumstances, may serve any or all of these roles.[1,2] Long-term successful management usually depends on identifying the possible contributing factors and is often proportionate to the thoroughness and accuracy of the initial assessment. Thus, a comprehensive diagnostic approach requires clinicians to understand all potential contributing factors relevant to TMD and chronic orofacial pain.

Many factors can affect the dynamic balance or equilibrium between the components of the masticatory system.[3] There are numerous factors driving the equilibrium either toward normal or adaptive physiologic health and function or toward dysfunction and pathology. Bone remodeling, TMJ soft tissue metaplasia, and muscle hypoactivity or hyperactivity are all adaptive physiologic responses to insult or change. Hyperactivity (hyperfunction) of the masticatory muscles, for example, from parafunction can affect the dynamic balance by biomechanically overloading the system contributing to long-term adaptive reactions.[3] Loss of structural integrity, altered function, or biomechanical overloading in the system can compromise adaptability and increase the likelihood of dysfunction or pathology. Direct extrinsic trauma to any component of the masticatory system can spontaneously initiate loss of structural integrity and concomitant altered function thereby reducing the adaptive capacity in the system. In addition, there are other contributing anatomic, systemic pathophysiologic, and psychosocial factors that may sufficiently reduce the adaptive capacity of the masticatory system and cause TMD.

Trauma

At this time, there is evidence to support trauma as an etiologic factor for a subset of TMD. In fact, overt trauma and adverse loading from parafunction may cause injury to the masticatory structures and are often implicated as etiologic factors leading to TMD signs and systems. Overt trauma that produces injury to the head, neck, or jaw can result from an impact injury.[4-6] An injury while eating, yawning, singing, or from prolonged mouth opening or extensive stretching, as may occur during long dental appointments, may lead to or aggravate TMD signs or symptoms. According to Pullinger and Seligman[7,8] 38% to 79% of adults in different diagnostic groups have a history of trauma compared to only 12% to 18% of nonpatients. Another study reported that a physical event was found in half the number of patients with nonreducing disc displacement, compared with only 27% in the muscle disorder group.[9] Katzberg et al[10] reported trauma as a cause of TMJ pain in 26% of pediatric TMD patients. Blows and abuse involving being struck in the mandible by a fist or an object precipitating TMJ noise and pain occur more often in women than in men.[11] Sports injuries including glancing or direct blows in contact sports can initiate TMD most often in the age range of 15 to 30 years. Iatrogenic trauma includes routine dental procedures such as extraction of teeth and cementation of crowns and fixed protheses especially on the mandibular arch.[4] Oral intubation for the administration of general anesthesia has also been implicated as an etiologic factor.[12]

Hyperextension injury with no direct blow to the face is suggested as a possible cause of TMD.[6,13] There is some evidence that TMD signs and symptoms are higher with hyperextension-flexion injury than in a noninjury controlled population,[6] but a direct causal relationship has yet to be established.[14] Braun et al[6] have emphasized that most of the evidence in hyperextension-flexion injuries is anecdotal. Thus, the condition of mandibular sprain at the time of a motor vehicular accident, without a direct blow to the mandible, resulting in hyperextension of the mandibular capsule, ligaments, and masticatory muscles is questionable.[5,14] Studies have shown that some patients with TMD have a cervical trauma history prior to the onset of TMD.[6] However, some of these studies do not separate cervical hyperextension-hyperflexion injuries from other forms of cervical trauma and the specific effects of this type of injury on the TMJ are not discussed. This is an area of uncertainty in which much misinformation is being provided to attorneys and patients without scientific studies to support the claims. This area is in need of clinical study and research.

Another form of trauma has been hypothesized to originate from sustained and repetitive adverse loading of the masticatory system through postural imbalances or from oral and parafunctional habits. It has been suggested that postural habits such as forward head position or phone-bracing may create muscle and joint strain and lead to musculoskeletal pain, including headache, in the TMD patient.[15]

Parafunctional habits such as teeth clenching, tooth grinding, lip biting, and abnormal posturing of the jaw are common and usually do not result in TMD symptoms. However, parafunctional habits have been suggested as initiating and/or perpetuating factors in certain subgroups of TMD patients.[16–27] The available research and clinical observations generally support this assumption; however, the exact role of parafunctional habits in TMD remains somewhat unclear because few studies have directly assessed these behaviors. Experimentally induced parafunction has been shown to cause pain similar to that reported by patients with TMD.[28,29] The intensity and frequency of parafunctional jaw activity may be exacerbated by stress and anxiety, sleep disorders, and medications (neuroleptics, alcohol, and other substances)[26]; and intense and persistent parafunction can occur in patients with neurologic disorders, such as cerebral palsy, and extrapyramidal disorders, such as orofacial dyskinesia and epilepsy.[30]

Parafunctional habits have been most frequently assessed by indirect means such as self-report, questionnaires, reports by a sleeping partner, or tooth wear. These indirect measures of parafunctional habits have provided conflicting reports as to the relationship between TMD symptoms and the presence of parafunctional habits. The limitations of these measures have recently been noted by Marbach et al.[31] Continued research with more direct measurements of parafunction, ie, portable electromyography, sleep laboratory, and direct observation, will be necessary to clarify the specific role of parafunction.

Anatomic Factors

Anatomic factors comprise maladaptive biomechanical relationships that can be genetic, developmental, or iatrogenic in origin. Severe skeletal malformations, interarch and intra-arch discrepancies, and past injuries to the teeth are examples of possible structural factors.

The dental profession historically has viewed malocclusion as a primary etiologic factor for TMD. Occlusal features such as working and nonworking posterior contacts and discrepancies between the retruded contact position (RCP) and intercuspal position (ICP) have been commonly identified as predisposing, initiating, and perpetuating factors. However, reviews of the literature and recent studies do not strongly support the role of anatomic etiologic factors.[32–41] Skull studies[42–44] and studies of patients with osteoarthrosis[45–50] have correlated loss of molar support with TMJ osteoarthrosis. However, the incidence of both osteoarthrosis and tooth loss increases with age and, when age is controlled, the associations vanish.[51] Studies of living nonpatient populations do not provide evidence of an association between TMD and lost molar support.[52–59] Further, a literature review did not reveal substantial evidence that moderate changes (approximately 4 to 6 mm) in occlusal vertical dimension (OVD) cause masticatory muscle hyperactivity or TMD symptoms.[60] Although occlusal guidance has been mentioned as influential for TMD signs and symptoms,[21] the majority of studies have not provided evidence for this association.[32,61–65]

Extensive overbite (vertical overlap of anterior teeth) was associated with joint sounds[62] and broad masticatory muscle tenderness,[66] but most studies do not support these associations.[63,65,67–73] Reduced overbite, in particular skeletal anterior open bite, however, has been associated with osteoarthrosis,[46,74,75] and with rheumatoid arthritis.[45,46]

Extensive overjet (horizontal overlap of anterior teeth) is mentioned as associated with TMD symptoms[67,71] and osteoarthrosis,[74] but other studies fail to provide evidence of overjet associations to TMD.[37,62,63,65,68–70,72,73,76–78] Recently, however, Seligman and Pullinger[40] have shown that overjet greater than 5 mm is very uncommon in a healthy nonpatient population.

Crossbite per se is not associated with TMD.[37,39,62,70,72,76,79–81] However, while a recent study has not found any evidence that anterior or posterior bilateral crossbite is associated with TMD, unilateral maxillary posterior lingual crossbite was found to be more common in TMD patients.[40]

There is a suggestion that those occlusal factors that are more prevalent in patients (large overjet, minimal overbite and anterior skeletal open bite, unilateral posterior crossbite, occlusal slides greater than 2 mm, lack of firm posterior tooth contact) are possibly the result of condylar positional changes following intracapsular alterations associated with disease but are not the cause of the disease.[40] However, examination of isolated occlusal factors, the valuative technique in the vast majority of past studies, is artificial and misleading and no doubt partially accounts for past confusion. Furthermore, whether considered individually or simultaneously, little evidence is available that occlusal and other associated factors that are traditionally implicated in TMD etiology (ie, Angle malocclusions, deep overbite, minimal overjet, severe attrition, anterior and bilateral posterior crossbite, condyle position, discrepancy between RCP and ICP, and unilateral RCP contacts) merit that association. Thus, studies to date suggest that occlusion is likely to be of secondary importance as a factor, exacerbating symptoms once TMD has become established for other reasons. Future scientifically controlled longitudinal epidemiologic studies are required to validate a relationship between occlusion and TMD.

Pathophysiologic Factors

All pathophysiologic factors primarily reflect systemic conditions and generally should be managed by the patient's primary physician or other medical specialist. These can include degenerative, endocrine, infectious, metabolic, neoplastic, neurologic, rheumatologic, and vascular disorders. These factors can act simultaneously on a central and local level.[82,83] The interacting tissues may be nonadjacent and dissimilar. For example, degenerative muscle changes can result from intracapsular disease.[84] It has been suggested that alterations in synovial fluid viscosity and inadequate lubrication may initiate clicking and derangement of the TMJ.[85] Synovial fluid analyses have attempted to correlate biochemical signs of inflammation with pain revealing abnormal concentrations of plasma proteins.[86,87] Other studies have evaluated the degradation of various enzymes, other metabolic by-products, as well as the type of pain transmitters causing pain, inflammation, and degeneration in the TMJ.[88,89]

Joint laxity has been cited as a possible contributing factor to TMD.[90,91] Systemic joint laxity has been shown to be significantly more prevalent in patients with articular disorders than with other TMD or with normal controls. Also, systemic joint laxity is significantly more prevalent in female than male adolescents.[92] Research has yet to demonstrate that the differences in populations can predict the potential of TMD.[93] Furthermore, physiologic response appears to be variable and individual.[94]

Of great concern to the diagnostician is the distinction between pathologic and adaptive responses to disease. Histologic studies suggest that cartilage thickness is a response to functional loading[95–98] and usually smooths radiographically observed bony irregularities through articular-surface soft tissue remodeling.[99,100] Even when cartilage was absent, loss of the fibrous connective-tissue covering of the articular bone was not observed. Thus, maintenance of an intact articular surface is to be expected, even in the face of osteoarthrosis.[57] This allows for both postural stability and histologic compatibility between the articulating components. Morphologic change, therefore, while mostly irreversible, usually achieves and maintains stability and should be considered adaptive. The proper goal of treating arthrosis in this light should not be to restore normal morphology but to encourage the body's adaptive response to pathophysiologic processes.

Psychosocial Factors

Psychosocial factors include individual, interpersonal, and situational variables that impact the patient's capacity to function adaptively. As a group, TMD and orofacial pain patients are significantly dissimilar both culturally and economically so the relevant psychosocial factors present with tremendous diversity. However, individual TMD patients may have personality characteristics or emotional conditions that make managing or coping with life situations difficult.[35,41,101–105] There is evidence that some patients with TMD experience more anxiety than do healthy control groups and that the TMD symptoms may be only one of several somatic manifestations of emotional distress.[106–108] These patients often have a history of other stress-related disorders.[109] Depression and anxiety related to other major life events may alter the patient's perception of and tolerance for physical symptoms, causing them to seek more care.[24,105,110,111] Chronic TMD patients have been found to have psychosocial and behavioral characteristics similar

to patients with lower back pain and headache.[112] However, one recent study found that TMD patients were not significantly different from other pain patients or healthy controls in personality type, response to illness, attitudes toward health care, or ways of coping with stress.[113]

It is important to note that anxiety and depression may not only result from and predispose patients to TMD, but that patients may present with mental disorders unrelated to TMD.[114,115] Mental disorders are syndromes of psychologic or organic origin that impair adaptive functioning in areas of emotion, perception, cognition, behavior, and/or interpersonal adjustment. The clinical features of mental disorders have been outlined by the American Psychiatric Association's DSM-IIIR.[116] Diagnostic criteria for psychotic syndromes, mood disturbances, anxiety disorders, organic mental disorders, and somatoform disorders are described. Somatization disorders, conversion disorders, psychogenic pain disorders, hypochondriasis, and atypical somatoform disorders are classified among the somatoform disorders. While the relationship of mental disorders to TMD awaits research documentation, clinical reports suggest that the psychologic conflicts and emotional distress of pre-existing psychiatric conditions may contribute to the etiology and exacerbation of or be intensified in response to TMD conditions.[117–119]

Environmental contingencies can greatly complicate treatment by affecting an individual's perception of and responses to pain and disease. Some patients may experience a lessening of distress to the extent that psychogenic symptoms decrease or resolve pre-existing psychologic and interpersonal conflicts. This *primary gain* of symptom formation is to be distinguished from the *secondary gain* of social benefits experienced by patients once a disorder is established.[120–123] Secondary gain includes being exempt from ordinary daily responsibilities, being compensated monetarily from insurance or litigation, using the rationalization of "being ill" to avoid unpleasant tasks, and gaining attention from family, friends, or health care workers.[124]

The use of alcohol, minor tranquilizers, narcotics, barbiturates, and other pharmaceuticals contributes substantially to the chronicity of many TMD patients. Every clinical assessment should pay careful attention to possible concurrent alcoholism or addiction in this patient group. The chemical dependency problems and pharmacologically induced depressions among TMD and chronic pain patients are frequently overlooked aspects that account for refractory responses to otherwise excellent treatment approaches.

Thus, psychosocial factors may predispose certain individuals to TMD and may also perpetuate TMD once symptoms have become established. A careful consideration of psychosocial factors is therefore important to the diagnostic evaluation and treatment of every TMD patient.

References

1. McNeill C: Craniomandibular (TMJ) disorders—the state of the art. Part II: Accepted diagnosis and treatment and modalities. J Prosthet Dent 1983;49:393–397.

2. McNeill C, Danzig WM, Farrar WB, Gelb H, Lerman MD, Moffett BC, Pertes R, Solberg WK, Weinberg LA: Craniomandibular (TMJ) disorders—The state of the art. Position Paper of The American Academy of Craniomandibular Disorders. J Prosthet Dent 1980;44:434–437.

3. Parker MW: A dynamic model of etiology in temporomandibular disorders. J Am Dent Assoc 1990;120:283–289.

4. Harkins SJ, Marteney JL: Extensive trauma: A significant precipitating factor in temporomandibular dysfunction. J Prosthet Dent 1985:271–272.

5. Burgess J: Symptom characteristics in TMD patients reporting blunt trauma and/or whiplash injury. J Craniomandib Disord Facial Oral Pain 1991;5:251–257.

6. Braun BL, Di Giovanna A, Schiffman E, Bonnema J, Fricton J: A cross-sectional study of temporomandibular joint dysfunction in post-cervical trauma patients. J Craniomandib Disord Facial Oral Pain 1992;6:24–31.

7. Pullinger AG, Seligman DA: TMJ osteoarthrosis: A differentiation of diagnostic subgroups by symptom history and demographics. J Craniomandib Disord Facial Oral Pain 1987;1:251–256.

8. Pullinger AG, Seligman DA: Trauma history in diagnostic groups of temporomandibular disorders. Oral Surg Oral Med Oral Pathol 1991;71:529–534.

9. Isacsson G, Linde C, Isberg A: Subjective symptoms in patients with temporomandibular joint disk displacement versus patients with myogenic craniomandibular disorders. J Prosthet Dent 1989;61:70–77.

10. Katzberg R, Tallents R, Hayakawa K, Miller T, Goske M, Wood B: Internal derangements of the temporomandibular joint: Findings in the pediatric age group. Radiology 1985;154:125–127.

11. Howard JA: Temporomandibular joint disorders, facial pain and dental problems of performing artists. In Sataloaff R, Brandfonbrener A, Lederman R (eds) Textbook of Performing Arts Medicine. New York, Raven Press Ltd, 1990, pp 111–169.

12. Taylor RC, Way WL: Temporomandibular joint problems in relation to the administration of general anesthesia. Oral Surg 1968;26:327–329.

13. Weinberg S, LaPointe H: Cervical extension-flexion injury (whiplash) and inter-

nal derangement of the temporomandibular joint. J Oral Maxillofac Surg 1987;45:653–656.

14. Goldberg HL: Trauma and the improbable anterior displacement. J Craniomandib Disord Facial Oral Pain 1990;4:131–134.

15. Travell JG, Simons DG: Myofascial Pain and Dysfunction: The Trigger Point Manual. Baltimore, Williams and Wilkins, 1983, pp 63–158.

16. Attanasio R: Nocturnal bruxism and its clinical management. Dent Clin North Am 1991;35:245–252.

17. Faulkner KDB: Bruxism: A review of the literature. Part I. Aust Dent J 1990;35:266–276.

18. Faulkner KDB: Bruxism: A reivew of the literature. Part II. Aust Dent J 1990;35:355–361.

19. Glaros AG, Rao SM: Effects of bruxism: A review of the literature. J Prosthet Dent 1977;38:149–157.

20. Graf H: Bruxism. Dent Clin North Am 1969;13:659–665.

21. Ingervall B, Mohlin B, Thilander B: Prevalence of symptoms of functional disturbances of the masticatory system in Swedish men. J Oral Rehabil 1980;7:185–197.

22. Laskin DM: Etiology of the pain dysfunction syndrome. J Am Dent Assoc 1969;79:147–153.

23. McGlynn FD, Cassisi JE, Diamond EL: Bruxism: A behavioral dentistry perspective. In Daitzman RJ (ed) Diagnosis and Intervention in Behavior Therapy and Behavioral Medicine. Vol 2. New York, Springer, 1985, pp 28–87.

24. Malow RM, Olson RE, Greene CS: Myofascial pain dysfunction syndrome: A psychophysiological disorder. In Golden C, Alcaparras S, Strider F, Graber B (eds) Applied Techniques in Behavioral Medicine. New York, Grune and Stratton, 1981, pp 101–133.

25. Nilner M: Relationship between oral parafunctions and functional disturbances in the stomatognathic system in 15 to 18 year olds. Acta Odontol Scand 1983;41:197–201.

26. Rugh JD, Harlan J: Nocturnal bruxism and temporomandibular disorders. Adv Neurol 1988;49:329–341.

27. Schärer P: Bruxism. In Kawamura Y (ed) Frontiers of Oral Biology. Basel, S Karger, 1974, pp 293–322.

28. Christensen L: Some effects of experimental hyperactivity of the mandibular locomotor system in man. J Oral Rehabil 1975;2:169–178.

29. Moss R, Ruff M, Sturgis E: Oral behavioral patterns in facial pain, headache, and non-headache populations. Behav Res Ther 1984;6:683–697.

30. Fahr S: The extrapyramidal disorders. In Cecil Textbook of Medicine. Vol 2. Philadelphia, WB Saunders Co, 1985, pp 2070–2077.

31. Marbach JJ, Raphael KG, Dohrenwend BP, Lennon MC: The validity of tooth grinding measures: Etiology of pain dysfunction syndrome revisited. J Am Dent Assoc 1990;120:327–333.

32. Bush FM: Malocclusion, masticatory muscle and temporomandibular joint tenderness. J Dent Res 1985;64:129–133.

33. DeLaat A, Van Steenberghe D, Lesaffre E: Occlusal relationships and TMJ dysfunction. Part II. Correlation between occlusal and articular parameters and symptoms of TMJ dysfunction by means of stepwise logistic regression. J Prosthet Dent 1986;55:116–121.

34. Droukas G, Lindee C, Carlsson GE: Occlusion and mandibular dysfunction: A clinical study of patients referred for functional disturbances of the masticatory system. J Prosthet Dent 1985;53:402–496.

35. Duinkerke AS, Luteijn F, Bouman TK, de Jong HP: Relations between TMJ pain dysfunction syndrome (PDS) and some psychologic and biographic variables. Community Dent Oral Epidemiol 1985;13:185–189.

36. Hannam AG, De Cou RE, Scott JD, Wood WW: The relationship between dental

occlusion, muscle activity and associated jaw movement in man. Arch Oral Biol 1977;22:25–32.

37. Pullinger AG, Seligman DA, Solberg WK: Temporomandibular disorders. Part II: Occlusal factors associated with temporomandibular joint tenderness and dysfunction. J Prosthet Dent 1988;59:363–367.

38. Pullinger AG, Seligman DA: Overbite and overjet characteristics of refined diagnostic groups of temporomandibular patients. Am J Orthod Dentofac Orthop 1991;100:401–415.

39. Seligman DA, Pullinger AG: Association of occlusal variables among refined TM patient diagnostic groups. J Craniomandib Disord Facial Oral Pain 1989;3:227–236.

40. Seligman DA, Pullinger AG: The role of intercuspal relationships in temporomandibular disorders: A review. J Craniomandib Disord Facial Oral Pain 1991;5:96–106.

41. Wänman A, Agerberg G: Etiology of craniomandibular disorders: evaluation of some occlusal and psychosocial factors in 19-year-olds. J Craniomandib Disord Facial Oral Pain 1991;5:35–44.

42. Granados J: The influence of the loss of teeth and attrition on the articular eminence. J Prosthet Dent 1979;42:78–85.

43. Whittaker DK, Davies G, Brown M: Tooth loss, attrition, and temporomandibular joint changes in a Romano-British population. J Oral Rehabil 1985;12:407–419.

44. Whittaker DK: Surface and form changes in the temporomandibular joints of 18th century Londoners. J Dent Res 1989;68 (special issue):abstr 1211.

45. Akerman S, Kopp S, Nilner M, Petersson A, Rohlin M: Relationship between clinical and radiologic findings of the temporomandibular joint in rheumatoid arthritis. Oral Surg Oral Med Oral Pathol 1988;66:639–643.

46. Tegelberg A, Kopp S: Clinical findings in the stomatognathic system for individuals with rheumatoid arthritis and osteoarthritis. Acta Odontol Scand 1987;45:65–75.

47. Kopp S: Clinical findings in temporomandibular joint osteoarthrosis. Scand J Dent Rest 1977;85:434–443.

48. Martinez M, Aguilar N, Barghi N, Rey R: Prevalence of TMJ clicking in subjects with missing posterior teeth. J Dent Res 1984;63(special issue):abstr 1568.

49. Barghi N, Aguilar CD, Martinez C, Woodall WS, Masskant BA: Prevalence of types of temporomandibular joint clicking in subjects with missing posterior teeth. J Prosthet Dent 1987;57:617–620.

50. Holmlund A, Helsing G, Axelsson S: The temporomandibular joint: A comparison of clinical and arthroscopic findings. J Prosthet Dent 1989;62:61–65.

51. Whittaker DK, Jones JW, Edwards PW, Molleson T: Studies on the temporomandibular joints of an eighteenth-century London population (Spitalfields). J Oral Rehabil 1990;17:89–97.

52. Pekkarinen V, Yli-Urpo A: Helkimo's indices before and after prosthetic treatment in selected cases. J Oral Rehabil 1987;14:35–42.

53. Helkimo M: Studies on function and dysfunction of the masticatory system. III: Analysis of anamnestic and clinical recordings of dysfunction with the aid of indices. Swed Dent J 1974;67:165–182.

54. Swanljung O, Rantanen T: Functional disorders of the masticatory system in southwest Finland. Community Dent Oral Epidemiol 1979;7:177–182.

55. Kirveskari P, Alanen P: Association between tooth loss and TMJ dysfunction. J Oral Rehabil 1985;12:189–194.

56. Wilding RJC, Owen CP: The prevalence of temporomandibular joint dysfunction in edentulous non-denture wearing individuals. J Oral Rehabil 1987;14:175–182.

57. Pullinger AG, Baldioceda F, Bibb CA: Relationship of TMJ articular soft tissue to underlying bone in young adult condyles. J Dent Res 1990;69:1512–1518.

58. Muir CB, Goss AN: The radiologic mor-

phology of asymptomatic temporomandibular joints. Oral Surg Oral Med Oral Pathol 1990;10:349–354.

59. Lundeen TF, Scruggs RR, McKinney MW, Daniel SJ, Levitt SR: TMJ symptomatology among denture patients. J Craniomandib Disord Facial Oral Pain 1990;4: 40–46.

60. Rivera-Morales WC, Mohl ND: Relationship of occlusal vertical dimension to the health of the masticatory system. J Prosthet Dent 1991;65:547–553.

61. Balthazar Y, Ziebert G, Donegan S: Limited mandibular mobility and potential jaw dysfunction. J Oral Rehabil 1987;14: 569–574.

62. Runge ME, Sadowsky C, Sakols EL, BeGole EA: The relationship between temporomandibular joint sounds and malocclusion. Am J Orthodont 1989;96:36–42.

63. Solberg WK, Flint RT, Brantner JP: Temporomandibular joint pain and dysfunction. A clinical study of emotional and occlusal components. J Prosthet Dent 1972;28:412–427.

64. Butler JH, Folke LEA, Brandt CL: A descriptive survey of signs and symptoms associated with the myofascial pain dysfunction syndrome. J Am Dent Assoc 1975;90:635–639.

65. Roberts CA, Tallents RH, Katzberg RW, Sanchez-Woodworth RE, Espeland MA, Handleman SF: Comparison of internal derangements of the TMJ with occlusal findings. Oral Surg Oral Med Oral Pathol 1987;63:645–650.

66. Seligman DA, Pullinger AG, Solberg WK: Temporomandibular disorders. Part III: Occlusal and articular factors associated with muscle tenderness. J Prosthet Dent 1988;59:483–489.

67. Riolo ML, Brandt D, Ten Have TR: Associations between occlusal characteristics and signs and symptoms of TMJ dysfunction in children and young adults. Am J Orthod Dentofac Orthop 1987;92:467–477.

68. Shian YY: Incidence of temporomandibular disorders in teenagers of Taiwan. J Dent Res 1989;68(special issue):abstr 26.

69. Gunn SM, Woolfold BW, Faja BW: Malocclusion and TMJ symptoms in migrant children. J Dent Res 1987;65(special issue):abstr 1174.

70. Cachiotti D, Plesh O, Bianchi P, McNeill C: Signs and symptoms in samples with and without temporomandibular disorders. J Craniomandib Disord Facial Oral Pain 1991;5:167–172.

71. Helöe B, Heiberg AN, Krogstad BS: A multiprofessional study of patients with myofascial pain-dysfunction syndrome I. Acta Odontol Scand 1980;38:109–117.

72. Helöe B, Helöe LA: Characteristics of a group of patients with temporomandibular joint disorders. Community Dent Oral Epidemiol 1975;3:72–79.

73. Pedersen A, Hansen H-J: Internal derangement of the temporomandibular joint in 211 patients: Symptoms and treatment. Community Dent Oral Epidemiol 1987;15:339–343.

74. Pullinger AG, Seligman DA: The degree to which attrition characterizes diagnostic groups of temporomandibular disorders. J Craniomandib Disord Facial Oral Pain (in press).

75. Williamson EH, Hall JT, Zwemer JD: Swallowing patterns in human subjects with and without temporomandibular dysfunction. Am J Orthod Dentofac Orthop 1990;98:507–511.

76. Lieberman MA, Gazit E, Fuchs C, Lilos P: Mandibular dysfunction in 10–18 year old school children as related to morphologic malocclusion. J Oral Rehabil 1985;12:209–214.

77. Castaneda R, McNeill C, Noble W: Biomechanical factors in TMJ osteoarthritis. J Dent Res 1988;67(special issue):abstr 87.

78. Castaneda R, McNeill C, Guerrero A: Biomechanics in TMJ osteoarthritis. Part II. J Dent Res 1989;68(special issue):abstr 620.

79. DeBoever JA, van den Berghe L: Longitudinal study of functional conditions in

the masticatory system in Flemish children. Community Dent Oral Epidermiol 1989;15:100–103.

80. Seligman DA, Pullinger AG, Solberg WK: Temporomandibular disorders. Part III: Occlusal and articular factors associated with muscle tenderness. J Prosthet Dent 1988;59:483–489.

81. Mohlin B, Kopp S: A clinical study on the relationship between malocclusion, occlusal interferences and mandibular pain and dysfunction. Swed Dent J 1978;2: 105–112.

82. Byrd KE, Stein ST: Effects of lesions to the trigeminal motor nucleus on temporomandibular disc morphology. J Oral Rehabil 1990;17:529–540.

83. Hagberg C, Hellsing G, Hagberg M: Perception of cutaneous electrical stimulation in patients with craniomandibular disorders. J Craniomandib Disord Facial Oral Pain 1990;4:120–125.

84. El-Labben NG, Harris M, Hopper C, Barber P: Degenerative changes in masseter and temporalis muscles in limited mouth opening and TMJ ankylosis. Oral Surg Oral Med Oral Pathol 1990;19:423–425.

85. Toller PA: The synovial apparatus and temporomandibular joint function. Br Dent J 1961;111:355–362.

86. Kopp S, Wenneberg B, Clemensson E: Clinical, microscopical and biochemical investigation of synovial fluid from temporomandibular joints. Scand J Dent Res 1983;91:33.

87. Israel HA: Synovial fluid analysis. Oral Maxillofac Surg Clin North Am 1989;1: 85–92.

88. Kakudo K: Ultrastructural cytochemical studies of horseradish peroxidase uptake by synovial lining cells of the rat temporomandibular joint. Okajima Folia Anat Jpn 1980;57:219–240.

89. Quinn JH, Bazan NG: Identification of prostaglandin E2 and leukotriene B4 in the synovial fluid of painful, dysfunctional temporomandibular joints. J Oral Maxillofac Surg 1990;48:968–971.

90. Hesse JR, Naeije M, Hansson TL: Craniomandibular stiffness towards maximum mouth opening in healthy subjects: A clinical and experimental investigation. J Craniomandib Disord Facial Oral Pain 1990;4:257–266.

91. Buchingham RB, Bruan T, Harinstein DA, Oral K et al: Temporomandibular joint dysfunction syndrome: A close association with systemic joint laxity (the hypermobile joint syndrome). Oral Surg Oral Med Oral Pathol 1991;72:514–519.

92. Westling L: Temporomandibular joint dysfunction and systemic joint laxity. Swed Dent J (Suppl 81) 1992.

93. Westling L, Carlsson GE, Helkimo M: Background factors in craniomandibular disorders with special reference to general joint hypermobility, parafunction, and trauma. J Craniomandib Disord Facial Oral Pain 1990;4:89–98.

94. Christensen LV, Donegan SJ: Observations in the time and frequency domains of surface electromyograms of experimental brief teeth clenching in man. J Oral Rehabil 1990;17:473–486.

95. Hansson T, Öberg T: Arthrosis and deviation in form in the temporomandibular joint. A macroscopic study on a human autopsy material. Acta Odontol Scand 1977;35:167–174.

96. Hansson T, Öberg T, Carlsson GE, Kopp S: Thickness of the soft tissue layers and the articular disk in the temporomandibular joint. Acta Odontol Scand 1977; 35:77–83.

97. Hansson T, Nordström B: Thickness of the soft tissue layers and articular disk in temporomandibular joints with deviations in form. Acta Odontol Scand 1977;35:281–288.

98. Lubsen CC, Hansson TL, Nordström BB, Solberg WK: Histomorphometric analysis of cartilage and subchondral bone in mandibular condyles of young human adults at autopsy. Arch Oral Biol 1985;30: 129–136.

99. Baldioceda F, Pullinger AG, Bibb CA: Relationship of condylar bone profiles and

dental factors to articular soft-tissue thickness. J Craniomandib Disord Facial Oral Pain 1990;4:71–79.

100. Baldioceda F, Bibb CA, Pullinger AG: Distribution and histologic character of osseous concavities in mandibular condyles of young adults. J Craniomandib Disord Facial Oral Pain 1990;4:147–153.

101. Rugh JD, Solberg WK: Psychological Implications in Temporomandibular Pain and Dysfunction. In Zarb GA, Carlsson GE (eds) Temporomandibular Joint Function and Dysfunction. Copenhagen, Munksgaard, 1979, pp 239–258.

102. Eversole LR, Stone CE, Matheson D, Kaplan H: Psychometric profiles and facial pain. Oral Surg Oral Med Oral Pathol 1985;60:269–274.

103. Harness DM, Rome HP: Psychological and behavioral aspects of chronic facial pain. Otolaryngol Clin North Am 1987; 22:1073–1094.

104. Southwell J, Deary IJ, Geissler P: Personality and anxiety in temporomandibular joint syndrome patients. J Oral Rehabil 1990;17:239–243.

105. Flor H, Birbawner N, Schulte W, Roos R: Stress-related electromyographic responses in patients with chronic temporomandibular pain. Pain 1991;46:145–152.

106. Gerschman JA, Wright JL, Hall WD, Reade PC, Burrows GD, Holwill BJ: Comparisons of psychological and social factors in patients with chronic orofacial pain and dental phobic disorders. Aust Dent J 1987;32(5):331–335.

107. Knutsson K, Hasselgren G, Nilner M, Petersson A: Craniomandibular disorders in chronic orofacial pain patients. J Craniomandib Disord Facial Oral Pain 1989; 3:15–19.

108. McCreary CP, Clark GT, Merril RL, Flack V, Oakley ME: Psychological distress and diagnostic subgroups of temporomandibular disorder patients. Pain 1991;44:29–34.

109. Gold S, Lipton J, Marbach J, Gurion B: Sites of psychophysiological complaints in MPD patients: II. Areas remote from the orofacial region. J Dent Res 1975;54 (special issue):abstr 165.

110. Molin C, Edman G, Schalling D. Psychological studies of patients with mandibular pain dysfunction syndrome. Swed Dent J 1973;66:15–23.

111. Melzack R: Neurophysiological Foundations of Pain. In Sternback RA (ed) The Psychology of Pain. 2nd ed. New York, Raven Press, 1986, pp 1–25.

112. Turk DC, Rudy TE: The robustness of an empirically derived taxonomy of chronic pain patients. Pain 1990;43:27–35.

113. Schnurr RF, Brooke RI, Rollman GB: Psychological correlates of temporomandibular joint pain and dysfunction. Pain 1990;42:153–165.

114. Gamsa A: Is emotional disturbance a precipitator or a consequence of chronic pain? Pain 1990;42:183–195.

115. Reisine ST, Weber J: The effects of temporomandibular joint disorders on patients' quality of life. Community Dent Health 1987;6:257–270.

116. American Psychiatric Association: Diagnostic and Statistical Manual. 3rd ed, revised. Washington, DC, American Psychiatric Association Press, 1987.

117. Bridges RN, Goldberg DP: Somatic presentation of DSM-III psychiatric disorders in primary care. J Psychosom Res 1985;29:563–569.

118. Lipowski ZJ: Somatization: The concept and its clinical application. Am J Psychiatry 1988;145:1358–1368.

119. Morrison J, Herbstein J: Secondary affective disorder in women with somatization disorder. Compr Psychiatry 1988;29:433–440.

120. Mechanic D: The concept of illness behavior: Culture, situation and personal predisposition. Psychol Med 1986;16:1–7.

121. Pilowsky I: Abnormal illness behavior. Br J Med Psychol 1969;42:347–351.

122. Pilowsky I, Smith QP, Katsikitis M: Illness behavior and general practice utilization:

A prospective study. J Psychosom Res 1987;31:177–183.

123. Wooley SC, Blackwell B, Winget C: A learning theory model of chronic illness behavior: Theory, treatment and research. Psychosom Med 1978;40:379–401.

124. Fordyce WE: Behavioral Methods for Chronic Pain and Illness. St Louis, CV Mosby, 1976.

Diagnostic Classification

Diagnostic Process

The first well-known classification of headache was proposed by the Ad Hoc Committee on Classification of Headache (AHCCH)[1] of the National Institute of Neurological Diseases and Blindness. This classification provided general guidelines for categorizing headaches based on clinical symptomatology. Because of shortcomings in the AHCCH system, the International Headache Society (IHS) established a committee in 1987 to reclassify headaches. This committee developed more specific criteria to provide greater uniformity and reproducibility in headache diagnosis. This system was published as the first edition of *Classification and Diagnostic Criteria for Headache Disorders, Cranial Neuralgias and Facial Pain* (see Flowchart).[2] This was the first major attempt to reclassify headache syndromes since the AHCCH's criteria were published in 1962. The American Academy of Orofacial Pain (AAOP), formerly the American Academy of Craniomandibular

Disorders (AACD) has collaborated with these organizations to include TMD in the diagnostic classification.[3]

A TMD classification system that is integrated with an existing medical diagnostic classification system facilitates communication and shared responsibility among dentists, physicians, and allied health care providers. Because of the multitude of disease entities that present with similar pain patterns in the head and neck region, dentists must consider diseases unrelated to the masticatory system in their differential diagnosis. Likewise, physicians evaluating craniofacial pain must also consider odontogenic pain and TMD in their differential diagnosis.

The diagnostic process is a clinical skill in which both art and science are wed.[4] The goals of the process are to determine the primary and any secondary physical or mental diagnoses, the contributing factors, and the level of complexity of the patient's problem(s) including the prognosis(es).[5,6] A problem list that identifies conditions or problems that may be

International Headache Society

Classification for Headache Disorders, Cranial Neuralgias, and Facial Pain*

1. Migraine headache
2. Tension-type headache
3. Cluster headache and chronic paroxysmal hemicrania
4. Miscellaneous headaches, unassociated with structural lesion
5. Headache associated with head trauma
6. Headache associated with vascular disorders
7. Headache associated with nonvascular intracranial disorders
8. Headache associated with substances or their withdrawal
9. Headache associated with noncephalic infection
10. Headache associated with metabolic disorder
11. Headache or facial pain associated with disorder of cranium, neck, eyes, ears, nose, sinuses, teeth, mouth, or other facial or cranial structures
12. Cranial neuralgias, nerve trunk pain, and deafferentation pain
13. Headache not classifiable

Recommended Diagnostic Classification* for

11 Headache or facial pain associated with disorders of cranium, eyes, ears, nose, sinuses, teeth, mouth, or other facial or cranial structures

11.1 Cranial bones including mandible
11.2 Neck
11.3 Eyes
11.4 Ears
11.5 Nose and sinuses
11.6 Teeth and related oral structures
11.7 Temporomandibular joint
11.8 Masticatory muscles

* Cephalgia, vol 8, supplement 7, 1988, Norwegian University Press, Publications Expediting Inc, or PO Box 2459 Tolyen 0609 Oslo 6, Norway.

** Adapted from American Academy of Craniomandibular Disorders, C. McNeill (ed): Craniomandibular Disorders: Guidelines for Evaluation, Diagnosis, and Management. Chicago, Quintessence Publ Co, 1990.

Recommended Diagnostic Classification** for

11.1 Cranial bones including the mandible
- **11.1.1 Congenital and developmental disorders**
  - 11.1.1.1 Aplasia
  - 11.1.1.2 Hypoplasia
  - 11.1.1.3 Hyperplasia
  - 11.1.1.4 Dysplasia
- **11.1.2 Acquired disorders**
  - 11.1.2.1 Neoplasia
  - 11.1.2.2 Fracture

Recommended Diagnostic Classification** for

11.7 Temporomandibular joint disorders
- **11.7.1 Deviation in form**
- **11.7.2 Disc displacement**
  - 11.7.2.1 Disc displacement with reduction
  - 11.7.2.2 Disc displacement without reduction
- **11.7.3 Dislocation**
- **11.7.4 Inflammatory conditions**
  - 11.7.4.1 Synovitis
  - 11.7.4.2 Capsulitis
- **11.7.5 Arthritides**
  - 11.7.5.1 Osteoarthrosis
  - 11.7.5.2 Osteoarthritis
  - 11.7.5.3 Polyarthritides
- **11.7.6 Ankylosis**
  - 11.7.6.1 Fibrous
  - 11.7.6.2 Bony

Recommended Diagnostic Classification** for

11.8 Masticatory muscle disorders
- **11.8.1 Myofascial pain**
- **11.8.2 Myositis**
- **11.8.3 Spasm**
- **11.8.4 Protective splinting**
- **11.8.5 Contracture**
- **11.8.6 Neoplasia**

responsible for each of the presenting complaints of the patient, as well as other factors that may contribute to the complexity of the tentative diagnoses, usually facilitates the process. The diagnostic process involves ruling out specific disorders from a diagnostic classification that includes all possible disorders that can cause similar symptoms. It is important to rule out serious, life-threatening intracranial or extracranial disorders or diseases early in the diagnostic process as these conditions may require immediate care. Attention is then directed toward odontogenic, TMD, and other sources of pain until the correct diagnosis(es) is(are) established using inclusive diagnostic criteria. The process of differential diagnosis is critical because an incorrect or omitted diagnosis is one of the most frequent causes of treatment failure.

Establishing the correct diagnosis in patients with chronic TMD and orofacial pain is particularly difficult because of the complex interrelationship of somatic and psychosocial factors in the etiology of chronic pain syndromes. Many disorders in this category have similar signs and symptoms and there is a high frequency of multiple diagnoses. If the source of painful symptoms is uncertain, the appropriate diagnosis is "pain, cause unknown or undetermined." Although individual clinicians are successful in diagnosing the more simple TMD problems, a team approach is often required for diagnosing and managing complex chronic TMD problems, especially when psychologic disorders may be present.[7] To facilitate this approach, Dworkin[8] suggested a multiaxial diagnostic system that develops concurrent physical, mental, and social conditions into two axes. Axis I includes the TMD clinical diagnoses, and axis II provides assessment and classification of nonpathophysiologic components of TMD pain conditions in terms of pain intensity, pain-related disability, depression, and nonspecific physical symptoms.

Differential Diagnosis of Orofacial Pain

Orofacial pain can be associated with pathology or disorders related to intracranial and extracranial structures (including TMD) and neurovascular, neuropathic, and psychogenic pain disorders (Fig 4-1).

Intracranial and Extracranial Structures

Disorders of the intracranial structures, eg, neoplasm, aneurysm, abscess, hemorrhage or hematoma, and edema should be considered first in the differential diagnosis because they can be life threatening and may require immediate attention. The characteristics of serious intracranial disorders include new or abrupt onset of pain or progressively more severe pain, interruption of sleep by pain, and pain precipitated by exertion or positional change (ie, coughing, sneezing). Also, weight loss, ataxia, weakness, fever with pain, and neurologic signs or symptoms (eg, seizure, paralysis, vertigo) and neurologic deficits are characteristic of intracranial disorders.[9] Besides masticatory structures and TMD, other extracranial structures and disorders should also be suspected as the source of orofacial pain. This includes disorders of the dental pulp, periodontium, mucosa, tongue, salivary glands, lymph tissues, sinuses, eyes, ears, nose, and throat. When doubt exists about a specific diagnosis, consultation with an appropriate specialist is essential.

Neurovascular Disorders

Neurovascular disorders associated with orofacial pain include migraine headache,

---

Differential Diagnosis of Orofacial Pain

Intracranial structures
- Neoplasm, aneurysm, abcess, hemorrhage, hematoma, edema

Extracranial structures
- Temporomandibular disorders, other craniofacial disorders, cervical disorders

Neurovascular disorders
- Migraine, migraine variants, cluster headache, paroxymal hemicrania, cranial artertis, carotidynia

Neuropathic pain disorders
- Paroxysmal neuralgias
  Trigeminal, glossopharyngeal, nervus intermedius, superior laryngeal neuralgias
- Continuous pain disorders
  Deafferentation pain syndromes (peripheral neuritis, postherpetic neuralgia, posttraumatic and postsurgical neuralgia)
- Sympathetic maintained pain

Psychogenic pain disorders
- Psychotic syndromes, mood disturbances, anxiety disorders, organic disorders, somatoform disorders

---

Fig 4-1 The diagnostic process involves ruling out specific disorders that may be responsible for each of the presenting complaints of the patient. From a diagnostic classification this includes disorders of the intracranial and extracranial structures, neurovascular disorders, neuropathic pain disorders, and psychogenic pain disorders.

migraine variants, cluster headaches, cranial arteritis, and carotidynia. The usual description of *vascular pain* is a throbbing, pulsating, or beating pain. Migraine headaches can be subdivided into migraine with aura (classic) and migraine without aura (common migraine). Migraine with aura headaches characteristically are one-sided and have a prodromal vasoconstriction phase with visual aberrations. This is followed by vasodilation of the affected arteries resulting in throbbing (pulsating) pain lasting 4 to 72 hours with frequently accompanying nausea and/or vomiting and phonophobia and photophobia.[10] Migraine without aura headaches are similar to classic migraines, but proceed into a headache without prodromata. At least five attacks are required as a diagnos-

tic criterion to separate migraine without aura from episodic tension-type headache. The site of pain in migrainous headaches is most frequently in the orbital, frontal, or temporal regions, but facial migrainous headaches also occur. The term *mixed muscular-vascular* (combination) *headache* is being eliminated in favor of both migraine and tension-type headache being individually coded for patients with coexisting conditions.[2] However, recently a vascular-supraspinal-myogenic model for pain in migraine has been proposed based on the theory that headache intensity is determined by the sum of nociception from cephalic arteries and pericranial myofascial tissues converging on the same neurons and integrated with supraspinal effects (usually facilitating) of somatovisceral afferents on nucleus caudalis neurons.[11] Migraine with aura variants include ophthalmoplegic, retinal, basilar, and hemiplegic migraines. Ophthalmoplegic and hemiplegic migraines are severe variations of classic migraine. The symptoms are accompanied by ocular motor nerve palsy and/or partial or complete paralysis of motor function. Retinal migraine is described as repeated attacks of monocular scotoma or blindness lasting less than an hour.

Cluster headache, also known as Horton's headache or histaminic neuralgia, and chronic paroxysmal hemicrania are similar to migrainous pain but are much more intense and of shorter duration than is migraine pain. The pain is usually reported as unilateral, excruciating, throbbing pain behind the eyes that occurs in clusters of days to weeks with periods of remission of months to years. The headaches can be provoked by alcohol, histamine, or nitroglycerine. Cluster headache frequently presents characteristic autonomic effects, ie, nasal congestion, lacrimation, conjunctival injection, edema of the eyelids and face on the affected side, that are commonly referred to as Horner's syndrome.[12,13] Cluster headaches are 10 to 50 times less common than are migraine headaches and are found at least 5 to 6 times more frequently in men than in women.[14] Chronic paroxysmal hemicrania are similar to cluster headaches but they are shorter lasting, more frequent, occur mostly in women, and remit immediately in response to indomethacin administration.

Headaches associated with other vascular disorders that can be related to orofacial pain include *cranial arteritis* and *carotidynia*. Cranial arteritis (temporal arteritis) is a giant-cell inflammatory disease of the carotid artery system (vasculitis) and is rarely seen in people under 50 years of age. The problem can easily be misdiagnosed as a muscular disorder when the temporal artery is involved. The danger of delayed diagnosis is that when there is involvement with the ophthalmic artery, subsequent blindness can occur. Carotidynia is a vascular disorder characterized by throbbing pain in the distribution of the external carotid artery, usually in the neck and face.[15] Palpation of the artery may reproduce the symptoms and project ipsilateral pain to the head. Other headaches that can resemble migraine headaches may be related to many different causes of vasodilation with associated throbbing pain (ie, altitude sickness, overexertion, dehydration, dialysis, certain allergens, caffeine, alcohol, and certain chemicals).

Neuropathic Pain Disorders

Neuropathic pain disorders can be divided into two main categories of painful conditions: paroxysmal and continuous.[16] The paroxysmal conditions causing orofacial pain include trigeminal neuralgia, glossopharyngeal neuralgia, nervous intermedius neuralgia, and superior laryngeal neuralgia.[17] Occipital neuralgia is not listed because the characteristic pain is located in the back of the cranium above the nuchal line rather than in the orofacial region. The common paroxysmal pain attack follows a distinct unilateral course and is described as electric-like, stabbing, or shooting pain. Attacks occur intermittently lasting for seconds to minutes with remissions for days, months, or even years. Stimulation of a trigger zone within the distribution of the affected nerve sets off a volley of pain attacks. *Trigeminal neuralgia* (tic douloureux) commonly involves the maxillary and/or mandibular division of the fifth cranial nerve which causes pain in the area of the distribution of either division of the trigeminal nerve.[18] *Glossopharyn-*

geal neuralgia is less common than is trigeminal neuralgia. Cutaneous trigger points are less common but, if present, are localized around the ear. Ordinary functions like coughing, chewing, swallowing, and talking may trigger pain. The pain is generally located in the ear, tonsillar area, throat, and pharynx.[19] *Nervus intermedius* (geniculate) *neuralgia* is rare and is described as a lancinating "hot poker" in the ear.[20] The trigger area is usually in the external auditory canal. *Superior laryngeal neuralgia* is also a rare disorder characterized by severe pain in the lateral aspects of the throat, submandibular region, and underneath the ear, precipitated by swallowing, shouting, or turning the head.[2]

The continuous neuropathic pain disorders associated with orofacial pain are primarily *deafferentation pain syndromes* (peripheral postherpetic neuralgia, posttraumatic and postsurgical neuralgia) and *sympathetically maintained pain conditions*. The pain is usually described as a persistent, ongoing, unremitting burning sensation. Patients frequently report abnormal sensations (dyesthesias) that are exacerbated by movement or touch. Deafferentation pain can occur as a result of inflammation, compression, distortion, demyelination, infarction, or paralysis of a nerve trunk. Referred pains and other central excitatory effects do not occur.[21] One common neuropathic pain condition, postherpetic neuralgia, is usually a constant, intense, unilateral burning pain with hyperesthesia that occurs after clearing of the herpes zoster virus from a peripheral nerve or dorsal root ganglion.[22] Posttraumatic and postsurgical (anesthesia dolorosa) neuralgias are described as a continuous tingling, numbness, twitching, or prickly sensation. This deafferentation pain results from damage to the nerve by trauma or surgery. The term *causalgia* has been used in the past for deafferentation

pain initiated by trauma of a major peripheral nerve.[23] Because disruption of the normal pathway that connects the neural elements of the dental pulp to the central nervous system occurs routinely with pulp extirpation during endodontic procedures and dental extraction, deafferentation is an important consideration in the differential diagnosis of unrelenting odontogenic pain.

Sympathetically maintained pain refers to a specific group of painful disorders precipitated by an injury to peripheral tissues and sustained by neural mechanisms that include sympathetic efferent activity.[24] The existence of this condition has been unequivocally demonstrated by sympathetic blockade (stellate ganglion block) producing immediate and complete relief of pain.[25] There appears to be some evidence that atypical odontalgia may be a sympathetically maintained pain.[26] The term *reflex sympathetic dystrophy* has been used when the sympathetically maintained pain is accompanied by progressive autonomic dysfunction, ie, changes in cutaneous temperature, color, texture, and perspiration followed by trophic changes in the skin, muscle, and bone.[27]

Psychogenic Pain Disorders

Stressful life events, such as conflicts in home or work relationships, financial problems, and cultural readjustment may contribute to illness and chronic pain.[28,29] These stressors may heighten tensions, insecurities, and dysphoric effects that may in turn lead to increased adverse loading of the masticatory system as psychic "stress," which is converted to muscle "tension" and increased parafunctional behaviors. Once established, these adjustment reactions (often with mixed disturbance of emotions and conduct) can further exacerbate the physical condition in a reverberating circuit of somatopsychic-psychosomatic problems.[30,31]

Depression, anxiety, and prolonged negative feelings are common among chronic pain patients and may make the persistent pain more difficult to tolerate or manage.[28,32] Individuals who unconsciously tend toward somatic expressions of emotions and conflicts are thought to be at higher risk of developing psychogenic somatic symptoms, including TMD, through increased autonomic nervous system arousal, chronic muscle tension, and neuroendocrinologic activation.[33,34] Negative cognitive factors, such as counterproductive thoughts or attitudes, can make resolution of the illness more difficult.[35,36] Confusion and misunderstanding are commonly seen in chronic pain patients because they often have received many opposing and varied opinions, diagnoses, and treatment suggestions. This confusion reduces motivation and increases anger or noncompliance. Also, patients with persistent pain often have unrealistic expectations and may expect complete or immediate pain relief.[32]

It is to be emphasized that mental disorders and TMD are not mutually exclusive conditions.[37] On the one hand, individuals with psychiatric disturbances may have bonafide TMD. Conversely, the lack of clear organic findings in patients with persistent symptoms of TMD is insufficient to impute a psychogenic origin to these complaints. The diagnosis of psychogenic pain requires the presence of specific signs and symptoms and should never be based on the exclusion of organic disease alone. When psychosocial factors are prominent in the patient's presentation, collaboration with a mental health professional should be an integral dimension of assessment and management.[38]

Diagnostic Classification System for TMD

Defining most TMD that produce musculoskeletal pain and dysfunction has been difficult due to the lack of clear etiologic factors and knowledge regarding the natural progression of TMD, as well as the lack of homogeneity of the patient population. However, as previously mentioned, the American Academy of Orofacial Pain has developed a well-defined diagnostic classification for TMD that is to be added to the Classification and Diagnostic Criteria for Headache Disorders, Cranial Neuralgias and Facial Pain by the International Headache Society (IHS).[3] This effort will help to emphasize the role of TMD in headache and orofacial pain. With the TMD diagnostic classification integrated within the existing medical diagnostic system, it is hoped that more accurate differential diagnoses can be established. However, some confusion still exists, particularly in distinguishing the muscle pain disorders (tension headache, mixed muscular-vascular headache, myofascial pain, fibromyalgia, and masticatory muscle disorders).[39]

Temporomandibular disorders are listed in the diagnostic classification of the IHS under the 11th major classification, namely, headache or facial pain associated with disorders of the cranial bones, neck, eyes, ears, nose, sinuses, teeth, mouth, or other facial or cranial structures (see Flowchart). Temporomandibular disorders are divided into disorders of the cranial bones including the mandible (IHS Classification 11.1), temporomandibular joint disorders (IHS Classification 11.7), and masticatory muscle disorders (IHS Classification 11.8). The International Classification of Diseases, 9th Revision, Clinical Modification Codes (ICD.9.CM), required by medical insurance, are given for each specific TMD.[40]

Disorders of the Cranial Bones and Mandible

Disorders of the cranial bones and mandible include *aplasia* (agenesis), *hypoplasia*, *hyperplasia*, *dysplasia*, *neoplasia*, and *fracture* (see Flowchart). Lesions and disorders of the jaws can be of either odontogenic or nonodontogenic origin and can be of generalized or metastatic nature. Most disorders of the cranial bones and mandible are congenital or developmental disorders and are rarely accompanied by orofacial pain. They are primarily disorders that cause problems with esthetics or function. Acquired disorders such as neoplasia (eg, osteomyelitis, multiple myeloma, Pagets' disease) and mandibular fracture can be a source of pain.

Congenital or Developmental Disorders

Aplasia (ICD.9.CM 754.0) Aplasia is a faulty or incomplete development of the cranial bones or mandible. Almost all aplasia of the mandible belong to the group of anomalies commonly known as hemifacial microsomia or first and second branchial arch syndromes. The most common developmental defect is the lack of growth of the condyle, usually resulting from incomplete development of the primordium of the condyle embryologically; in this case there is little to no articular fossa and a rudimentary or absent eminence. The auditory apparatus is frequently affected. The complete congenital absence (agenesis) of the mandible or maxilla is extremely rare.[41]

Hypoplasia (ICD.9.CM 526.89) Hypoplasia is the incomplete development or underdevelopment of cranial bones or mandible that is congenital or acquired. The growth is considered to be normal although proportionately reduced. It is less severe in degree than is aplasia. Many craniofacial anomalies include incomplete development of the cranial bones and mandible, eg, Treacher-Collins syndrome.[42] Condylar hypoplasia can be secondary to trauma.

Hyperplasia (ICD.9.CM 526.89) Hyperplasia is the overdevelopment of the cranial bones or mandible, which can be congenital or acquired. It is a nonneoplastic increase in the number of normal cells. It can occur as a localized enlargement, ie, condylar hyperplasia or coronoid hyperplasia, or as an overdevelopment of the entire mandible or side of the face.[43] Excessive size of the mandible is termed mandibular prognathism, which results in protrusion of the chin with no abnormality of condylar size, shape, or function.

Dysplasia (ICD.9.CM 526.89) Fibrous dysplasia is a benign slow-growing swelling of the mandible and/or maxilla characterized by the presence of fibrous connective tissue[44] with a characteristic whorled pattern and containing trabeculae of immature nonlamellar bone.[45] Radiographically the lesion may appear varied, from an opaque ground-glass to a lucent appearance, depending on the ratio of fibrous tissue to bone. There is usually no displacement of teeth, the cortical bone remains intact, and the occlusion of the dental arches remains undisturbed. The disease occurs particularly in children and young adults and usually becomes inactive when they reach skeletal maturity.

Acquired Disorders

Neoplasia (ICD.9.CM 213.1 [benign]; 170.1 [malignant]) Neoplasia is a new, abnormal, and uncontrolled growth of the cranial bones or mandible. Neoplasia includes benign, malignant, and metastatic tumors. Benign tumors, ie, osteoma, chondroma, osteoblastoma, chondroblastoma, ameloblastoma, and synovial chondromatosis are most commonly found in the TMJ. Malignant tumors, ie, osteosarcoma, Ewing's sarcoma, chondrosarcoma, fibrosarcoma, adenocarcinoma do exist but are exceedingly rare. Approximately 1% of malignant neoplasia metastasize to the jaws.[46,47]

Fracture (ICD.9.CM 802.21 [condylar process]) Extrinsic traumatic force can injure all related bony components of the masticatory system (ie, temporal bone, maxilla, zygoma, sphenoid bone, and mandible) possibly causing the following: fracture, dislocation, contusion, and/or laceration of articular surfaces, ligaments, and disc, with or without hemarthrosis intraarticularly. Sequelae could include adhesions, ankylosis, or joint degeneration.[48]

Joint Disorders

Temporomandibular joint disorders can be divided into articular disorders related to *deviation in form, articular disc displacement, dislocation, inflammatory conditions, arthritides,* and *ankylosis*[3] (see Flowchart). These subclassifications are similar to disorders in other synovial joints in the body even though the articular surfaces of the temporomandibular joint are covered with noninnervated, avascular fibrous connective tissue as opposed to hyaline cartilage.

Deviation in Form (ICD.9.CM 524.69)

Deviation in form is described as painless mechanical dysfunction or altered function due to irregularities or aberrations in form of intracapsular soft and hard articular tissues. It can occur because of developmental or acquired conditions, which include physiologic remodeling related to adverse loading.[49,50] When a developmental process causes an anatomic deviation in form or an acquired remodeling process causes a loss of integrity in the articular surfaces, a mechanical interference clinically manifested as joint sounds on function may result. The condition is nonpainful and the resultant asymptomatic joint sounds usually occur at the same

condylar positions on opening and closing of the mandible.[51]

Diagnostic criteria

1. Complaint of faulty or compromised joint mechanics (eg, joint noise, intermittent locking, or dislocation)
2. Reproducible joint noise usually at same position during opening and closing mandibular movements
3. Radiographic evidence of mild structural bony abnormality or loss of normal shape may also exist

Disc Displacement (ICD.9.CM 524.63)

Articular disc displacement is the most common TMJ arthropathy and is characterized by several stages of clinical dysfunction that involve the condyle-disc relation. It is characterized by an abnormal relation or misalignment of the articular disc and condyle.[52–56] Although posterior[57] and mediolateral[58–60] displacements of the articular disc have been described, the usual direction for displacement is in an anterior or anteromedial direction.[61,62] The causes of disc displacement are not agreed upon; however, it is postulated that in a majority of cases the disc is permitted to be displaced by stretched or torn ligaments that bind the disc to the condyle.[63] A recent study associated an increased horizontal angle of the mandibular condyle and internal derangement of the TMJ. The condylar angle was increasingly larger with more advanced pathologic changes.[64] Disc displacement is subdivided into disc displacement with reduction or disc displacement without reduction.

Disc Displacement With Reduction Disc displacement with reduction is described as an abrupt alteration or interference of the disc-condyle structural relation during mandibular translation with mouth opening and closing. From a closed mouth position the "temporarily" misaligned disc reduces or improves its structural relation with the condyle when mandibular translation occurs with mouth opening, which produces a joint noise (sound) described as clicking or popping. Disc displacement with reduction usually is characterized by what is termed *reciprocal clicking*, a reciprocal noise that is heard during the opening movement and again just before the teeth occlude during the closing movement. The closing noise is usually of less magnitude and is thought to be produced by the displacement, once again, of the disc. The momentary jamming or misalignment of the disc has been theorized to be due to articular surface irregularity, disc-articular surface adherence, synovial fluid degradation, disc-condyle incoordination as a result of abnormal muscle function, increased muscle activity across the joint, or disc deformation. Because disc displacement with reduction is so common, it is reasonable to consider the disorder as a physiologic adaptation that develops an important equilibration of force distribution and does not necessarily represent a pathologic response.[65–68] Thus, TMJ dysfunction (asymptomatic clicking) itself does not warrant treatment.[69]

Pain, if present, is precipitated by joint movement and usually occurs at the time of the disc reduction. Painful disc displacement with reduction is thought to be due to gross injury that results in stretching or tearing of the disc ligaments and/or capsule of the joint. As the condition becomes more chronic or as the disc becomes further displaced, it begins to interfere later in the translating (opening) movement. Previously used terms for this condition include internal derangement, anterior disc displacement, reciprocal disc, and disc-condyle incoordination.

Diagnostic criteria

1. Pain, when present, is precipitated by joint movement.

2. Reproducible joint noise occurs usually at variable positions during opening and closing mandibular movements.

3. Soft tissue imaging reveals displaced disc that improves its position during jaw opening.

Disc Displacement Without Reduction

Disc displacement without reduction is described as an altered or misaligned disc-condyle structural relation that is maintained during mandibular translation. Thus, the disc is nonreducing or "permanently" displaced and does not improve its relation with the condyle on translation; in fact, the relation may become worse. It sometimes is referred to as a "closed lock". When acute, it is usually painful and is characterized by sudden and marked limited jaw motion because of a jamming or fixation of the disc secondary to disc adhesion, deformation, and/or dystrophy.[70] It is manifested clinically as a straight line deviation to the affected side on opening, a marked limited laterotrusion to the contralateral side, and a lack of joint noise. Disc displacement without reduction is often associated with overt trauma and, when acute, the accompanying pain is exacerbated by function. As the condition becomes chronic, the pain is markedly reduced from the acute stage to the point of becoming nonpainful in many cases, and the opening range may approach normal dimensions over time. If chronic, there usually is a history of joint noise and/or limitation of mandibular opening.[71,72]

Diagnostic criteria (acute)

1. Pain precipitated by function.

2. Marked limited mandibular opening.

3. Straight line deviation to the affected side on opening.

4. Marked limited laterotrusion to the contralateral side.

5. Soft tissue imaging reveals displaced disc without reduction.

Diagnostic criteria (chronic)

1. Pain, when present, is markedly reduced from acute stage.

2. History of joint noise and/or limitation of mandibular opening.

3. Slight limited mandibular opening, if at all.

4. Slight limited laterotrusion to the contralateral side.

5. Soft tissue imaging reveals displaced disc without reduction.

Dislocation (ICD.9.CM 830.1 [open])

Temporomandibular joint dislocation, also known as *open-lock* or *subluxation*, describes a condition in which the condyle is positioned anterior to the articular eminence and is unable to return to a closed position. It is manifested clinically as an inability to close the jaw. Dislocation may be the result of (1) a physical jamming of the disc-condyle complex beyond the articular eminence that is maintained by muscle activity; (2) a true hyperextension of the disc-condyle complex beyond its normal maximum translation position; or (3) failure of the disc to rotate about the condyle during jaw closure due to disc distortion and attachment elongation. The duration of dislocation can be prolonged and patients are only able to normalize jaw function with manipulation by a clinician. There usually is a clinical history of excessive range of motion that is not painful, but pain can occur at the time of dislocation with residual pain following the episode.

Diagnostic criteria

1. Inability to close the mandible.

2. Pain, if present, occurs at time of dislocation with mild residual pain after the episode.

3. Radiographic evidence reveals condyle well beyond the eminence.

Inflammation (ICD.9.CM 727.09)

Primary inflammatory conditions of the TMJ are relatively uncommon and are associated primarily with rheumatologic disease. Inflammatory conditions, including synovitis or capsulitis, frequently occur secondary to trauma, irritation, or infection and often accompany other TMJ disorders.[73] Synovitis is described as an inflammation of the synovial lining of the TMJ that can be due to infection, an immunologic condition secondary to cartilage degeneration, or trauma. Synovitis is characterized by localized pain that is exacerbated by function and superior and/or posterior joint loading. Many times there will be a fluctuating swelling (due to effusion) that decreases the ability to occlude on the ipsilateal posterior teeth. Capsulitis, an inflammation of the capsule related to sprain of capsular ligaments, is difficult, if not impossible, to differentiate from synovitis but may also exhibit pain on joint distraction. Previously used terms include arthritis, arthralgia, discitis, and retrodiscitis.

Diagnostic criteria

1. Localized pain at rest exacerbated by function, especially with superior and/or posterior joint loading.

2. Limited range of motion secondary to pain. When present, fluctuating swelling (due to effusion) decreases ability to occlude on ipsilateral posterior teeth. An MRI may give a bright signal if fluid is present (T2 weighting).

Arthritides

Arthritides of the TMJ include localized *osteoarthrosis*, *osteoarthritis*, and generalized *polyarthritides*.[74]

Osteoarthrosis (ICD.9.CM 715.38) Osteoarthrosis is defined as a degenerative, noninflammatory condition of the joint characterized by structural changes of the joint surfaces secondary to excessive strain in the remodeling mechanism.[75] The onset is insidious and usually not associated with systemic disease. Osteoarthrosis is no longer considered a part of aging or simply a wear-and-tear process. Some researchers believe that it is due to a physiologic imbalance between the stress applied to a joint and the ability of the physiologic "shock absorbers" — soft tissue, cartilage, and bone — to deal successfully with the stress of loading.[76,77] As degeneration occurs there is a deterioration and abrasion of the articular cartilage and remodeling of underlying bone.[78–80] The process accelerates as proteoglycan depletion, collagen fiber network disintegration, and fatty degeneration weaken the functional capacity of the articular cartilage. Previous terms commonly used were osteoarthritis, arthritis, degenerative joint disease, and arthrosis deformans. Osteoarthrosis is characterized clinically by an absence of pain, probable crepitus, and usually a limited range of motion and deviation to the affected side on opening secondary to degeneration.[81] At the later stages of osteoarthrosis there is radiographic evidence of structural bony changes; however, early cartilage degeneration would only be detectable with biopsy or possibly with arthroscopy.[63]

Diagnostic criteria

1. Crepitus
2. Limited range of motion causes deviation to the affected side on opening
3. Radiographic evidence of structural

bony change (subchondral sclerosis, osteophytic formation) and joint space narrowing

Osteoarthritis (ICD.9.CM 524.62 [arthralgia]) Osteoarthritis (OA) is a degenerative condition accompanied by secondary inflammation (synovitis) of the TMJ. Typically the disease is slowly progressive but OA can have remissions and cartilage regeneration[82] characterized by deterioration of the articular cartilage and secondary new bone formation. Osteoarthritis is frequently localized to the temporomandibular joint in question but may be a part of a generalized condition.[83,84] Clinical findings include point tenderness on palpation, crepitus, limited range of motion with deviation on opening to the affected side, and radiographic evidence of structural bony changes. The articular changes are associated with (1) external or overt jaw trauma, (2) repetitive adverse loading, (3) infection, or (4) an idiopathic degenerative process. Although coarse crepitus can be diagnostic, confirmation of the diagnosis is based on joint imaging and pain. One rare idiopathic degenerative condition termed condylysis occurs spontaneously, primarily in adolescent females.[85–87] Normal condylar development proceeds until the sudden lytic event occurs causing the condyle to become progressively smaller and in some cases even disappear. Condylysis is not usually associated with ankylosis, erosive changes in the fossae, or a positive serologic test.

Diagnostic criteria

1. Pain with function due to the inflammation
2. Point tenderness on palpation
3. Crepitus or multiple joint noises
4. Limited range of motion with deviation on opening to the affected side

5. Radiographic evidence of structural bony change (subchondral sclerosis osteophytic formation) and joint space narrowing

Polyarthritides **(ICD.9.CM 714.9 [unspecified])** Joint inflammation and structural change caused by a generalized systemic polyarthritic condition are referred to as *polyarthritides*. Temporomandibular joint polyarthritides include rheumatoid arthritis, juvenile rheumatoid arthritis (Still's disease), spondyloarthropathies (ankylosing spondylitis, psoriatic arthritis, infectious arthritis, Reiter's syndrome), and crystal-induced disease (gout, hyperuricemia). Other rheumatologically related diseases that may affect the TMJ include autoimmune disorders and other mixed connective tissue diseases (scleroderma, Sjögren's syndrome, lupus erythematosus).[70] Polyarthritides are characterized by pain during acute and subacute stages, possible crepitus, limited range of motion secondary to pain and/or degeneration, and bilateral radiographic evidence of structural bony changes. This group of arthritides comprises multiple diagnostic categories that are best diagnosed with the aid of serology and managed by rheumatologists. Dental management relates to secondary complaints. Bilateral resorption of condylar structures can result in an anterior open bite in many cases.

Diagnostic criteria

1. Pain during acute and subacute stages
2. Point tenderness on palpation during acute stage
3. Crepitus
4. Limited range of motion secondary to pain and/or degeneration
5. Radiographic evidence of structural bony change

(Anterior open bite and abnormal serology findings may also be present.)

Ankylosis (ICD.9.CM 524.61)
Ankylosis is defined as a restricted mandibular movement with deviation to the affected side on opening that often results as a long-term sequela of trauma including mandibular fracture.[88] It implies a firm, unyielding restriction due to either intra-articular fibrous or bony ankylosis and is not associated with pain. Fibrous adhesions within the TMJ are thought to occur mainly in the superior compartment of the TMJ. They produce a decreased movement of the disc-condyle complex. Adhesions can occur secondary to joint inflammation that results from external trauma or systemic conditions such as a polyarthritic disease. Bony ankylosis results from the union of the bones of the TMJ by proliferation of bone cells; this causes complete immobility of that joint. No radiographic findings other than absence of ipsilateral condylar translation on opening are found with fibrous ankylosis. Bony ankylosis is characterized by radiographic evidence of bone proliferation with marked deviation to the affected side and marked limited laterotrusion to the contralateral side.

Diagnostic criteria (fibrous)

1. Limited range of motion on opening
2. Marked deviation to the affected side
3. Marked laterotrusion to the contralateral side
4. Radiographic findings that reveal absence of ipsilateral condylar translation on opening

Diagnostic criteria (bony)

1. Extreme limited range of motion on opening when condition is bilateral

2. Marked deviation to the affected side when condition is unilateral

3. Marked limited laterotrusion to the contralateral side when condition is unilateral

4. Radiographic evidence of bone proliferation and absence of condylar translation

Masticatory Muscle Disorders

Masticatory muscle disorders are analogous to muscle disorders that can occur in other areas of the head, neck, body, and extremities. They include myofascial pain, myositis, spasm, protective splinting, contracture, and neoplasia[3] (see flowchart). The mechanisms that cause pain to originate in skeletal muscles are still not well understood. Overuse of a normally profused muscle or ischemia of a normally working muscle may cause pain.[89–91] Sympathetic and fusimotor reflexes can produce changes in the blood supply and muscle tone; furthermore, different psychologic or emotional states can alter muscle tone. Neurons that mediate pain from skeletal muscle are subject to strong modulatory influences. The nociceptive endings can be sensitized very easily by endogenous substances (bradykinin, serotonin, prostaglandin [PGE$_2$], neuropeptides and substance P). These painful muscle conditions not only result in increased sensitivity of peripheral nociceptors, but also produce hyperexcitability in the central nervous system.[90]

On examination the jaw-closing muscles of the large majority of TMD patients are tender to palpation and approximately 40% of TMD patients report pain on chewing.[92] Traditionally it has been hypothesized that these symptoms are associated with increased postural electromyographic (EMG) activity.[93] However, Lund and co-workers[94] have questioned the commonly held view that musculoskeletal pain is maintained by some form of tonic muscular hyperactivity. Their studies show that the activity of agonist muscles is often reduced by pain with small increases in the level of antagonist muscle activity. As a result, maximum voluntary contraction, force production, and the range and velocity of movement are often reduced.

Fibromyalgia, also termed myofascitis, myofibrositis, or fibrositis, is often confused with myofascial pain; however, it should not be considered a specific masticatory muscle disorder even though there may be concurrent masticatory muscle pain.[39] Fibromyalgia is manifested as a generalized, continuous, aching pain and is associated with tenderness in many sites over the body, sleep disturbances, and depression. It may also be associated with generalized fatigue, chronic headache, anxiety, subjective swelling, irritable bowel syndrome, and modulation of the symptoms by activity or the weather. Descriptors include pain in three of four quadrants for at least 3 months, tenderness in 11 of 18 specific spots, and association with normal EMG activity.[95–98]

Myofascial Pain (ICD.9.CM 729.1)
Myofascial pain is characterized by a regional, dull, aching pain and presence of localized tender spots (trigger points) in muscle, tendons, or fascia that reproduce pain when palpated and may produce a characteristic pattern of regional referred pain and/or autonomic symptoms on provocation.[99–102] Myofascial pain can be confused with muscle contraction headache or tension headache and previously used terms include myalgia, trigger-point pain, and myofascial pain dysfunction syndrome. Palpation of the "active" trigger points causes reproducible alteration of pain to a more extensive area that may or may not include the muscle containing

the trigger points.[103,104] Inactivation of the trigger-point area with injection of local anesthetics, ice, or vapocoolant spray followed by stretch or transcutaneous electrical nerve stimulation (TENS) relieves the larger area of pain. The pathogenesis of myofascial pain is not well understood. There is evidence that a localized ischemia may cause the characteristic trigger-point sensitivity. Recently, interest has focused on the central nervous system, including the sympathetic nervous system, as a mediator of myofascial pain.

Diagnostic criteria

1. Regional pain, usually dull
2. Localized tenderness in firm bands of muscle and/or fascia
3. Reduction in pain with local muscle anesthetic injection or vapocoolant spray to trigger point followed by stretch

(A reproducible alteration of pain complaints with palpation at specific tender areas may also occur.)

Myositis (ICD.9.CM 728.81)

Myositis is usually due to local causes such as infection or injury. To help explain the clinical variations in painful muscle conditions, the term myositis is divided into two types of inflammatory responses. The first condition, which is primarily theoretical, is referred to as a painful condition due to intermittent overuse that results in interstitial inflammation and is referred to as delayed onset muscle soreness. There is no swelling, increased EMG activity, or trigger points and referral of pain with delayed onset muscle pain. The second condition is referred to as an extensive, clinically recognizable, inflamed muscle.

The second type of myositis is a constant, acutely painful, generalized inflammation and swelling, usually of the entire muscle. Because chemical substances produced in response to tissue damage and inflammation are presumably the principal cause of pain, elevated serum enzyme levels should be found; conversely, with interstitial inflammation without muscle cell damage there is no rise in serum enzyme levels.[90] Clinically, the patient may exhibit a limited range of motion. Ossification of a muscle can occur secondary to inflammation, which results in myositis ossificans. The inflammation may occur in the tendinous attachments of the muscle as well; this type of inflammation is termed either tendinitis or tendomyositis.

Diagnostic criteria (delayed onset muscle soreness)

1. Increased pain with mandibular movement
2. Onset following prolonged or unaccustomed use (up to 48 hours afterward)

Diagnostic criteria (generalized myositis)

1. Pain, usually acute, in localized area
2. Localized tenderness over entire region of the muscle
3. Increased pain with mandibular movement
4. Moderately to severly limited range of motion due to pain and swelling
5. Onset following injury or infection

Myospasm (ICD.9.CM 728.85)

Myospasm (acute trismus or cramp) is an acute disorder and is an involuntary, sudden, tonic contraction of a muscle. A muscle in spasm is acutely shortened, grossly limited in range of motion, and painful. Spasm is a continuous muscle contraction (fasciculation) and can, therefore, be differentiated from protective muscle splinting by needle or fine wire

EMG verification of sustained involuntary muscle contraction even at rest.[105,106]

Diagnostic criteria

1. Acute pain
2. Continuous muscle contraction (fasciculation)
3. Increased EMG activity even at rest (as measured with fine wire EMG)

Protective Muscle Splinting (ICD.9.CM 728.89)

Protective muscle splinting is defined as restricted or guarded mandibular movement due to co-contraction of muscles as a means of avoiding pain caused by movement of the parts.[107] Protective splinting is a central-nervous-system-induced response characterized by a limited range of motion, rigidity of jaw on manipulation, and pain. This problem can be further differentiated into (1) protective splinting to avoid a painful dysfunction, such as painful TMJ clicking, or (2) traumatic trismus due to operative trauma or regional injury. Another type of reflex splinting due to behavioral factors is termed hysterical trismus, which is a severe restriction of mandibular motion due to acute psychologic distress.[108] Patients with protective splinting or trismus do not exhibit muscle contraction when the jaw is at rest.

Diagnostic criteria

1. Severe pain with function, but not at rest
2. Marked limited range of motion without significant increase on passive stretch

Contracture (ICD.9.CM 728.9)

Muscle contracture or physiologic rigor (chronic trismus, muscle fibrosis, or muscle scarring) is a chronic resistance of a muscle to passive stretch as a result of fibrosis of the supporting tendons, ligaments, or muscle fibers themselves. Muscle contracture is usually caused by trauma but can result from infection or any disorder that results in hypomobility. It is not painful in general. Experiments suggest that there is a close relation between lowered adenosine triphosphate (ATP) concentrations and the occurrence of contracture.[109]

Diagnostic criteria

1. Limited range of motion
2. Unyielding firmness on passive stretch
3. History of trauma or infection

Neoplasia (ICD.9.CM 171.0)

Masticatory muscle neoplasia is defined as a new, abnormal, or uncontrolled growth of muscle tissue. It can be malignant or benign and may or may not be associated with pain. A myxoma is an example of a muscle neoplasm.

References

1. Ad Hoc Committee on Classification of Headache. Classification of headache. JAMA 1962;179:717–718.

2. Olesen J: Classification and Diagnostic Criteria for Headache Disorders, Cranial Neuralgias and Facial Pain. Cephalgia, An International Journal of Headache. 1988, Oslo, Norway, Norwegian University Press; 1988, Vol 8, Suppl 7.

3. American Academy of Craniomandibular Disorders: McNeill (ed) Craniomandibular Disorders: Guidelines for Evaluation, Diagnosis, and Management. Chicago, Quintessence Publ Co, 1990.

4. Harrison T: Principles of Internal Medicine. 11th ed. New York, McGraw-Hill Publ Co,1987, pp 1–15.

5. Carlsson GE: Mandibular dysfunction in temporomandibular joint pathosis. J Prosthet Dent 1980;43:658–662.

6. Reynolds MO: Is the concept of temporomandibular pain dysfunction syndrome valid? J Craniomand Pract 1988;6:299–307.

7. Fricton JR, Hathaway KM: Interdisciplinary management: Address complexity with teamwork. In Fricton JR, Kroening RJ, Hathaway KM (eds) TMJ and Craniofacial Pain: Diagnosis and Management. St Louis, Ishiyaku, Euro-American, Inc, 1988, pp 167–172.

8. Dworkin SF: Research diagnostic criteria for temporomandibular disorders. Final project report. Dworkin SF (ed) NIDR Epidemiology and Oral Disease Prevention Program, 1992.

9. Fricton JR, Kroening RJ, Schellhas KP: Differential diagnosis, the physical disorder. In Fricton JR, Kroening RJ, Hathaway KM (eds) TMJ and Craniofacial Pain: Diagnosis and Management. St Louis, Ishiyaku, Euro-American, Inc, 1988, pp 53–65.

10. Edmeads JG: Migraine. J Craniomandib Disord Facial Oral Pain. 1987;1:21–25.

11. Olesen J: Clinical and pathophysiological observations in migraine and tension-type headache explained by integration of vascular, supraspinal and myofascial inputs. Pain 1991;46:125–132.

12. Raskin NH, Appenzeller O: Cluster headache. In Headache: Major Problems in Internal Medicine. Vol 19. Philadelphia, WB Saunders Co, 1980, pp 185–198.

13. Pearce JMS: Cluster headache and its variants. Headache Q 1991;2:187–191.

14. Campbell JK: Cluster headache. J Craniomandib Disord Facial Oral Pain 1987; 1:27–33.

15. Raskin NH, Prusiner S: Carotidynia. Neurology 1977;27:43–46.

16. Fields HL: Pain Syndromes in Neurology. Oxford, Butterworth Heinemann Ltd, 1990, pp 14–16.

17. Fricton JR, Kroening RJ: Neuralgic disorders: Peripheral nerve pain. In Fricton JR, Kroening RJ, Hathaway KM (eds), TMJ and Craniofacial Pain: Diagnosis and Management. St Louis, Ishiyaku, Euro-America Inc, 1988, pp 131–137.

18. Loeser JD: The management of trigeminal neuralgia. Pain 1977;3:155–162.

19. Stevens JC: Cranial Neuralgia. J Craniomandib Disord Facial Oral Pain 1987;1: 51–53.

20. Bruyn GW: Nervus intermedius neuralgia (Hunt). In Rose FC (ed) Headache. Handbook of Clinical Neurology. Amsterdam, Elsevier, 1986;4:487–494.

21. Bell WE: Orofacial Pains. Classification, Diagnosis, Management. 4th ed. Chicago, Year Book Medical Publ, 1989, pp 377–416.

22. Loeser JD: Herpes zoster and post-herpetic neuralgia pain. Pain 1986;25:149–164.

23. Bonica JJ: Causalgia and other reflex sympathetic dystrophies. In Bonica JJ (ed) Advances in Pain Research and Therapy. Vol 13. New York, Raven Press Ltd, 1979, pp 141–166.

24. Roberts WJ, Kramis RC: Sympathetic nervous system influence on acute and chronic pain. In Fields HL (ed) Pain Syndromes in Neurology. Oxford, Butterworth Heinemann Ltd, 1990, pp 85–106.

25. Fields HL: Pain. New York, McGraw-Hill Book Co, 1987; pp 145–158.

26. Graff-Radford SB, Solberg WK: Common Problems in Pain Management. Chicago, Yearbook Medical Publishers, 1990, pp 23–27.

27. Kroening RJ, Fricton JR: Neuralgic disorders and causalgia disorders. In Fricton JR, Kroening J, Hathaway KM (eds) TMJ and Craniofacial Pain: Diagnosis and Management. St Louis, Ishiyaku, Euro-American Inc, 1988, pp 131–141.

28. Dworkin SF, Burgess JA: Orofacial pain of psychogenic origin: Current concepts and classification. J Am Dent Assoc 1987;115: 565–571.

29. Rugh JD, Davis SE: Temporomandibular disorders: Psychological and behavioral aspects. In Sarnat BG, Laskin DM (eds) The Temporomandibular Joint: A Biological Basis for Clinical Practice. 4th ed. Philadelphia, WB Saunders Co, 1992, pp 329–345.

30. Barsky AJ, Klerman GL: Overview: Hypochondriasis, bodily complaints, and somatic styles. Am J Psychiatry 1983;140(3):273–283.

31. Lipowski ZJ: Stomatization: The concept and its clinical application. Am J Psychiatry 1988;145:1358–1368.

32. Rugh JD: Psychological components of pain. Dent Clin North Am 1987;31:579–594.

33. Gordon E, Kraiuhin C, Kelly P: A Neurophysiological study of somatization disorder. Compr Psychiatry 1986;27:295–301.

34. Mardsen CD: Hysteria—A neurologist's view. Br J Psychiatry 1986;16:277–288.

35. Lesser IM, Ford CV, Friedmann CTH: Alexithymia in somatizing patients. Gen Hosp Psychiatry 1979;1:256–261.

36. Ciccone DC, Grzesiak RC: Cognitive dimensions of chronic pain. Soc Sci Med 1984;19:1339–1345.

37. Quill TE: Somatization disorder. JAMA 1985;254:3075–3079.

38. Smith GR, Monson RA, Ray DC: Psychiatric consultation in somatization disorders. N Engl J Med 1986;314:1407–1413.

39. Rogers EJ, Rogers RJ: Tension-type headaches, fibromyalgia, or myofascial pain. Headache Q 1991;2:273–277.

40. US Department of Health and Human Services, International Classification of Diseases, 9th Revision, Clinical Modification. 4th ed. Washington DC, 1992.

41. Brecht K, Johnson CM: Complete mandibular agenesis. Report of a case. Arch Otolaryngol 1985;111:132–134.

42. Behrents RG, McNamara JA, Avery JK: Prenatal mandibulofacial dysostosis (Treacher-Collins Syndrome). Cleft Pal J 1977;14:13–34.

43. Ricketts RM: Cephalometric synthesis. Am J Orthod 1960;46:647–673.

44. Poswillo DE: Congenital malformations: Prenatal experimental studies. In Sarnat BG, Laskin DM (eds) The Temporomandibular Joint. 3rd ed. Springfield, Charles C. Thomas, 1979, pp 127–150.

45. Schajowicz F, Ackerman LV, Sissons AA, Sobin LH, Torloni H: Histological typing of bone tumours. Geneva, World Health Organization, 1972.

46. Rubin MM, Jui V, Cozzi GM: Metastatic carcinoma of the mandibular condyle presenting as temporomandibular joint syndrome. J Oral Maxillofac Surg 1989;47:507–510.

47. Aniceto GS, Penin AG, de la Meta Pages R, Moreno JJM: Tumors metastatic to the mandible. Analysis of nine cases and review of the literature. J Oral Maxillofac Surg 1990;48:246–251.

48. Bell WE: Temporomandibular Disorders. Classification, Diagnosis, Management. 3rd ed. Chicago, Year Book Medical Publ 1990, pp 113–114.

49. Moffett BC, Johnson LC, McCabe JB, Askew HC: Articular remodeling in the adult human temporomandibular joint. Am J Anat 1964;115:119–142.

50. Hansson TL: Temporomandibular joint anatomical findings relevant to the clinician. In Clark GT, Solberg WK (eds) Perspectives in Temporomandibular Disorders. Chicago, Quintessence Publ Co, 1987, pp 45–54.

51. Carlsson GE, Oberg T: Remodeling of the temporomandibular joints. Oral Sci Rev 1974;4:53–86.

52. Farrar WB: Differentiation of temporomandibular joint dysfunction to simplify treatment. J Prosthet Dent 1972;28:629–636.

53. Dolwick MF: Diagnosis and etiology of internal derangements of the temporomandibular joint. In Laskin D, Greenfield W, Gale E, et al (eds) The President's Conference on the Examination, Diagnosis and Management of Temporomandibular Joint Disorders. Chicago, Am Dent Assoc 1983, pp 112–117.

54. Juniper RP: The pathogenesis and investigation of TMJ dysfunction. Brit J Oral Maxillofac Surg 1987;25:105–112.

55. Sanchez-Woodworth RE, Tallents RH, Katzberg RW, Guay JA: Bilateral internal

derangements of the TMJ: Evaluation by MRI imaging. Oral Surg Oral Med Oral Pathol 1988;65:281–285.

56. Helms CA, Doyle GW, Orwig D, et al: Staging of internal derangements of the TMJ with magnetic resonance imaging: Preliminary observations. J Craniomandib Disord Facial Oral Pain 1989;3:93–99.

57. Blankestijn J, Boering G: Posterior dislocation of the temporomandibular disc. Int J Oral Surg 1985;14:437–443.

58. Khoury MD, Dolan E: Sideways dislocation of the temporomandibular joint meniscus: The edge sign. Am J Nucl Radiol 1986;7:869–872.

59. Westesson P-L, Kurita K, Ericksson L, Katzberg RW: Cryosectional observations of functional anatomy of the temporomandibular joint. Oral Surg Oral Med Oral Pathol 1989;68:247–251.

60. Liedberg J, Westesson P-L, Kurita K: Side-ways and rotational displacement of the temporomandibular joint disk: Diagnosis by arthrography and correlation to cryosectional morphology. Oral Surg Oral Med Oral Pathol 1990;69:757–763.

61. Isberg-Holm AM, Westesson P: Movement of the disc and condyle in temporomandibular joints with clicking: An arthrographic and cineradiographic study on autopsy specimens. Acta Odontol Scand 1982;40:151–164.

62. Farrar WB, McCarty WL Jr: A Clinical Outline of Temporomandibular Joint Diagnosis and Treatment. 7th ed. Montgomery, Normandie, 1982, pp 53–88.

63. Stegenga B: Temporomandibular joint osteoarthrosis and internal derangement: Diagnostic and therapeutic outcome assessment. Thesis. Gröningen, Netherlands, 1991.

64. Westesson P-L, Bifano JA, Tallents RH, Hatala MP: Increased horizontal angle of the mandibular condyle in abnormal temporomandibular joints: A magnetic resonance imaging study. Oral Surg Oral Med Oral Pathol 1991;72:359–363.

65. Scapino RP: Histopathology associated with malposition of the human temporomandibular joint disc. Oral Surg Oral Med Oral Pathol 1983;55:382–397.

66. Scapino RP: The posterior attachment: Its structure, function, and appearance in TMJ imaging studies. Part 1. J Craniomandib Disord Facial Oral Pain 1991;5:83–95.

67. Scapino RP: The posterior attachment: Its structure, function, and appearance in TMJ imaging studies. Part 2. J Craniomandib Disord Facial Oral Pain 1991;5:155–166.

68. Blaustein D, Scapino RP: Remodeling of the temporomandibular joint disk and posterior attachments in disk displacement specimens in relation to glycosaminoglycan content. Plast Reconstr Surg 1986;78:756–764.

69. Greene CS, Laskin DM: Long term status of TMJ clicking in patients with myofascial pain dysfunction. J Am Dent Assoc 1988;117:461–465.

70. Stegenga B, de Bont LGM, Boering G: A proposed classification of temporomandibular disorders based on synovial joint pathology. J Craniomand Pract 1989;7:107–118.

71. Eversole LR, Machado L: Temporomandibular joint internal derangements and associated neuromuscular disorders. J Am Dent Assoc 1985;110:69–79.

72. Nickerson JW, Boering G: Natural course of osteoarthrosis as it relates to internal derangement of the temporomandibular joint. Oral Maxillofac Surg Clin North Am 1989;1:27–45.

73. Schüle H: Injuries of the temporomandibular joint: Classification, diagnosis and fundamentals of treatment. In Krüger E, Schilli W (eds) Oral and Maxillofacial Traumatology. Vol 2. Chicago, Quintessence Publ Co, 1986.

74. Carlsson GE, Kopp S, Oberg T: Arthritis and allied diseases. In Zarb GA, Carlsson GE (eds) Temporomandibular Joint Function and Dysfunction. Copenhagen, Munksgaard, 1979, pp 269–320.

75. DeBont LGM, Boering G, Liem RSB, Havinga P: Osteoarthritis of the temporomandibular joint: A light microscopic and scanning electron microscopic study of the articular cartilage of the mandibular condyle. J Oral Maxillofac Surg 1985; 43:481–488.

76. Bland JH, Stulberg SD: Osteoarthritis: Pathology and clinical patterns. In Keeley WM et al (eds) Textbook of Rheumatology. 2nd ed. Philadelphia, WB Saunders Co, 1985.

77. Radin EL, et al: Mechanical aspects of osteoarthrosis. Bull Rheum Disord 1975; 26:862–865.

78. Kopp S: Clinical findings in temporomandibular joint osteoarthrosis. Scand J Dent Rest 1977;85:434–443.

79. Castelli WA, Nasjleti CE, Diaz-Perez R, Caffesse RG: Histopathologic findings in temporomandibular joints of aged individuals. J Prosthet Dent 1985;53:415–419.

80. Stegenga B, de Bont LGM, Boering G, Van Willigen JD: Tissue responses to degenerative changes in the temporomandibular joint: A review. J Oral Maxillofac Surg 1991;49:1079–1088.

81. Rasmussen OC: Clinical findings during the course of temporomandibular arthropathy. Scand J Dent Res 1981;89: 283–288.

82. Bland JH, Cooper SM: Osteoarthritis: A review of the cell biology involved and evidence for reversibility. Semin Arthritis Rheum 1984;14:106–133.

83. Blackwood HJJ: Arthritis of the mandibular joint. Br Dent J 1963;115:317–376.

84. Toller P: Osteoarthritis of the mandibular condyle. Br Dent J 1973;134–223.

85. Rabey GP: Bilateral mandibular condylysis—a morphanalytic diagnosis. Brit J Oral Surg 1977/1978;15:121–134.

86. Caplan HI, Benny RA: Total osteolysis of the mandibular condyle in progressive systemic sclerosis. Oral Surg 1978;46:362–366.

87. Lanigan DT, Myall RWT, West RA, McNeill RW: Condylysis in a patient with a mixed collagen vascular disease. Oral Surg 1979;48:198–204.

88. Block MS, Provenzano J, Neary JP: Complications of mandibular fractures. Oral Maxillofac Surg Clin North Am 1990; 2:525–550.

89. Layzer RB: Muscle pain, cramps, and fatigue. In Engel AG, Banker BQ (eds) Myology: Basic and Clinical, New York, McGraw-Hill Publ Co, 1986, pp 1907–1923.

90. Mense S: Physiology of nociception in muscles. In Fricton JR, Awad E (eds) Advances in Pain Research and Therapy. Vol 17. New York, Raven Press Ltd, 1990, pp 67–85.

91. Mense S: Considerations concerning the neurobiological basis of muscle pain. Can J Physiol Pharmacol 1991;69:610–616.

92. Dworkin SF, Huggins KH, Le Resche L, Von Korff M, Howard J, Truelove E, Sommers E: Epidemiology of signs and symptoms in temporomandibular disorders. Clinical signs in cases and controls. J Am Dent Assoc 1990;120:273–281.

93. Dahlstrom L, Carlsson SG, Gale EN, Jansson TG: Stress-induced muscular activity in mandibular dysfunction: Effect of biofeedback training. J Behav Med 1985;8:191–200.

94. Lund JP, Donga R, Widmer CG, Stohler CS: The pain-adaptation model: A discussion of the relationship between chronic musculoskeletal pain and motor activity. Can J Physiol Pharmacol 1991;69: 683–694.

95. Goldenberg DL: Clinical features of fibromyalgia. In Fricton JR, Awad EA (eds) Advances in Pain Research and Therapy. Vol 17. Myofacial Pain and Fibromyalgia. New York, Raven Press Ltd, 1990, pp 139–163.

96. Wolfe F, Smythe HA, Yunus MB, Bennett RM, Bombardier C, Goldenberg DL, Tugwell P: The American College of Rheumatology, 1990: Criteria for the classification of fibromyalgia. Arthritis Rheum 1990;33:160–172.

97. Bennett RM: Recognizing fibromyalgia. Patient Care, July 1989: pp 60–83.

98. Bennett RM: Etiology of the fibromyalgia syndrome: A contemporary hypothesis. Intern Med Specialist 1990;11:48–61.

99. Shiffman A. Myofascial pain associated with unilateral masseteric hypertrophy in a condylectomy patients. J Craniomand Pract 1984;2:373–376.

100. Clark GT: Muscle Hyperactivity, Pain and Dysfunction. In Klineberg I, Sesale B (eds) Orofacial Pain and Neuromuscular Dysfunction: Mechanisms and Clinical Correlates. Sydney, Pergamon Press, 1985, pp 103–111.

101. Solberg WK: Temporomandibular disorders: Masticatory myalgia and its management. Br Dent J 1986;160:351–356.

102. Fricton JR: Myofascial pain syndrome: Characteristics and epidemiology. In Fricton JR, Awad EA (eds) Advances in Pain Research and Therapy. Vol 17. Myofacial Pain and Fibromyalgia. New York, Raven Press Ltd, 1990, pp 107–127.

103. Travell JG, Simons DG: Myofascial Pain and Dysfunction: The Trigger Point Manual. Baltimore, Williams and Wilkins, 1983, pp 63–158.

104. Fricton J, Kroening R, Haley D, Siegert R: Myofascial pain syndrome of the head and neck: A review of clinical characteristics of 168 patients. Oral Surg Oral Med Oral Pathol 1982;60:615–623.

105. Layzer RB: Diagnostic implications of clinical fasiculations and cramps. In Rowland LP (ed) Human Motor Neuron Diseases. New York, Raven Press Ltd, 1982 pp 23–27.

106. Roth G: The origin of fasciculations. Ann Neurol 1982;12:542–547.

107. Tveteras K, Kristensen S: The aetiology and pathogenesis of trismus. Clin Otolaryngol 1986;11:383–387.

108. Revington PJ, Peacock TR, Kingscote AD: Temporomandibular joint dysfunction: A case of hysterical trismus. Br Dent J 1985;158:55–56.

109. Sahlin K, Eldstrom L, Sigholm H, Hultlman E: Effects of lactic acid accumulation and ATP decrease on muscle tension and relaxation. Am J Physiol 1981;240:C121–C126.

Assessment

Collection of baseline records and other diagnostic data is fundamental to the proper management of TMD. The extent to which any or all of the elements of evaluation are pursued depends on the magnitude of the presenting complaints and the potential for the problem to progress physically or psychosocially. However, it is important for all clinicians to realize that many clinical signs important in the differential diagnosis of specific TMD subsets are not measured with high reliability.[1] In particular, assessment of pain on muscle palpation and identification of specific TMJ sounds have only modest to marginal reliability.

A screening evaluation is appropriate for all routine dental patients; whereas a comprehensive evaluation, ie, history and physical examination, is needed for patients presenting with signs or symptoms suggestive of TMD. Radiographic studies and soft tissue imaging of the TMJ and associated structures may be necessary for evaluation of articular disorders. Further, patients suffering from chronic orofacial pain may require behavioral and psychosocial assessment. Occasionally, to confirm a clinical impression, additional diagnostic tests for a specific diagnosis may be required (such as diagnostic injections, biopsies, and hematologic testing).

Screening Evaluation

Screening for TMD is recommended as an essential part of the routine dental examination.[2] The screening consists of a questionnaire, brief history, and examination (Figs 5-1 and 5-2). The aim of screening is to determine the presence or absence of TMD signs and symptoms. If significant findings are identified and recorded, a comprehensive history taking and clinical examination should be conducted.[2,3]

Comprehensive History

The history should parallel the traditional medical history and review of systems.

Recommended Screening Questionnaire for TMD

1. Do you have difficulty, pain, or both when opening your mouth, for instance, when yawning?
2. Does your jaw get "stuck," "locked," or "go out"?
3. Do you have difficulty, pain, or both when chewing, talking, or using your jaws?
4. Are you aware of noises in the jaw joints?
5. Do your jaws regularly feel stiff, tight, or tired?
6. Do you have pain in or about the ears, temples, or cheeks?
7. Do you have frequent headaches and/or neckaches?
8. Have you had a recent injury to your head, neck, or jaw?
9. Have you been aware of any recent changes in your bite?
10. Have you previously been treated for a jaw-joint problem? If so, when?

Fig 5-1 All patients should be screened for TMD through a questionnaire that includes these questions. The decision to actually complete a comprehensive history and clinical exam will depend on the number of positive responses and the apparent seriousness of the problem for the patient, ie, a positive response to any question may be sufficient to warrant a TMD exam if it is a concern to the patient or is viewed as clinically important by the clinician.

A comprehensive history includes (1) identification of the chief complaint; (2) a history of the present illness; (3) a medical history; (4) a dental history; and (5) a personal history (Fig 5-3). The chief complaint(s) or the purpose of the patient's visit should be stated succinctly. The chief complaint is the one symptom that the patient states as the most bothersome and the one most desired to be changed. Because patient complaints are often numerous, they should be prioritized according to the patient's concerns. The history of the present illness is a narrative report of each symptom or complaint: date of onset, onset event, character, intensity, duration, frequency, location, remissions, change over time, modifying factors including those that alleviate, aggravate, or precipitate individual episodes of pain, and previous treatment results. Any interrelationships among symptoms should be noted. When neurologic signs or symptoms are present (eg, numbness, visual disturbances, dizziness, vertigo, fa-

cial paralysis, and/or cranial nerve deficits), it is critical to rule out intracranial pathology as the cause. Space-occupying lesions such as a tumor, hematoma, and arteriovenous malformation must be considered.

The relevant medical history may include previous surgeries, hospitalizations, traumas, illnesses, developmental and acquired anomalies, and medications used. Contributing factors also should be assessed. For instance, the quality of the patient's sleep pattern is important because it may relate to depression and musculoskeletal pain. The dental history should include previous dental disease, treatment, and attitude. A habit history also identifies potential contributing factors such as bruxism (clenching or grinding), repetitive chewing (eg, excessive gum chewing), and abnormal jaw and tongue postural habits (eg, nail biting and lateral tongue bracing).[3]

The personal history of TMD patients is important because it often identifies

---

Recommended Screening Examination Procedures for TMD

1. Measure range of motion of the mandible on opening and right and left laterotrusion. (Note any incoordination in the movements.)
2. Palpate for preauricular or intrameatal TMJ tenderness.
3. Auscultate and/or palpate for TMJ sounds (ie, clicking or crepitus).
4. Palpate for tenderness in the masseter and temporalis muscles.
5. Note excessive occlusal wear, excessive tooth mobility, buccal mucosal ridging, or lateral tongue scalloping.
6. Inspect symmetry and alignment of the face, jaws, and dental arches.

Fig 5-2 All patients should be screened for TMD using this or a similar cursory clinical examination. The need for a comprehensive history and clinical examination will depend on the number of positive findings and the clinical significance of each finding. Any one positive finding may be sufficient to warrant a TMD exam.

psychosocial contributing factors; however, many patients are hesitant to discuss fully their personal history. They may be reluctant to share information on previous or current psychiatric counseling, depression, anxiety, impaired social and occupational activities, pending litigation or disability claims, family relationships, and other personal matters. Open communication is necessary to complete the history and to ensure comprehensive treatment. If this proves difficult, either because the patient becomes very distressed or because the patient describes significant problems, consultation with a relevant mental health specialist must be considered.

Comprehensive Physical Examination

Physical examination for TMD consists of observation and documentation of a general inspection of the head and neck, an evaluation of the functional status of the TMJs and cervical spine, an evaluation of the masticatory and cervical muscles, a cursory neurovascular evaluation includ-

ing a sensory and motor evaluation of the cranial nerves, and an intraoral evaluation including an occlusal analysis[3] (Fig 5-4).

General Inspection of the Head and Neck

Inspection of the head and neck includes visual and manual inspection of each anatomic structure to help rule out tumors, infections, and other pathology. Clinicians should be aware of unusual asymmetry, size, color, consistency, shape, posture, involuntary movement, or tenderness that might suggest an infectious, edematous, neoplastic, degenerative, obstructive, or dysfunctional process.

Evaluation of the TMJ and Cervical Spine

Measure and record mandibular opening and lateral movements. Two vertical opening measurements are suggested: full active opening by the patient (unassisted) and range of motion with passive (assisted) stretch applied by the clinician. The localization of pain with active move-

---

Comprehensive History Format for TMD Patients

Chief complaint

History of present illness

Date and event of onset
Location of signs and symptoms
Character, intensity, duration, frequency of signs and symptoms
Remissions or change over time
Modifying factors (alleviate, precipitate, or aggravate)
Previous treatment results

Medical history

Current or pre-existing relevant physical disorders or disease (specifically systemic
    arthritides or other musculoskeletal/rheumatologic conditions)
Previous treatments, surgeries, and/or hospitalizations
Trauma (specifically to head, face, or neck)
Medications (prescription, nonprescription)
Allergies
Alcohol and other substances of abuse

Dental history

Current or pre-existing relevant physical disorders or disease
Previous treatments including patient's attitude toward treatment
History of trauma to the jaw, teeth, or supporting tissues (including iatrogenic trauma)
Parafunctional history, both diurnal and nocturnal

Personal history

Social, behavioral, and psychologic
Occupational, recreational, and family
Litigation, disability, or other secondary gain issues

Fig 5-3 The sequence of a comprehensive history should parallel the traditional medical history and review of systems format including the patient's chief complaint(s), the history of each complaint or present illness, medical and dental histories, and finally a personal history.

ment or passive stretching of the jaw and the quality and symmetry of jaw movements should be noted. Document the presence and location of audible joint sounds, palpable clicking, or interference with jaw movement. Any manipulated or altered jaw position that eliminates, alleviates, or aggravates the joint pain, sounds, or incoordination should be noted. Palpate the TMJ for tenderness and swelling over the lateral (pre-auricular) and posterior (intrameatal) aspects of the joint capsule in the closed mouth position and during condylar translation. The amount and type of joint end-feel should be evaluated and noted. Observe active range of head and cervical spine movement and note pain responses to extension, flexion, rotation and side bending movements. Evaluate cervical joint noises and neurosensory signs or symptoms in the neck and shoulders.

Masticatory and Cervical Muscle Evaluation

Tenderness, swelling, enlargement, and unusual texture are noted from palpation

---

Comprehensive TMD Physical Examination Procedures

General inspection of the head and neck

  Note unusual asymmetry, size, shape, color, consistency, posture, and involuntary movement or tenderness

Evaluation of the TMJ and cervical spine

  Palpate the TMJ preauricularly and intrameatally
  Measure range of motion, quality of movement, and association with pain
  Auscultate and/or palpate for joint noises in all movements
  Guide mandible movement noting pain, end feel, and joint noise.

Masticatory and cervical muscle evaluation

  Note tenderness, swelling, enlargement, and unusual texture

Neurovascular evaluation

  Vascular compression of temporal and carotid arteries
  Cranial nerve signs and symptoms

Intraoral evaluation

  Hard and soft tissue conditions or disease
  Occlusal analysis, both static and dynamic

Fig 5-4 Physical examination for TMD consists of observation and documentation of a general inspection of the head and neck, an evaluation of the functional status of the TMJs and cervical spine, an evaluation of the masticatory and cervical muscles, a neurovascular evaluation, and an intraoral evaluation including an occlusal analysis.

of the following masticatory muscles: temporalis, deep and superficial masseter, medial pterygoid, and suprahyoids. Recent studies confirm that an algometer or pain-threshold meter can be reliably used to measure muscle tenderness.[4–6] The same inspection of the following cervical muscles or muscle groups is performed: sternocleidomastoid, suboccipital, paravertebral (scalenus), posterior deep cervical, and upper trapezius. Evaluation of the cervical musculature, nerves, and spine is recommended due to the high percentage of orofacial pain patients who also have craniocervical disorders.[7–9] If further study of the cervical region is needed, a referral to an appropriate specialist is necessary.

Neurovascular Evaluation

Compression testing of the temporal and carotid arteries for pain provocation is important to rule out giant cell arteritis and carotidynia. Neuropathies of the cranial nerves are manifested as disturbances of smell, sight, hearing, equilibrium, taste, and response to touch on the face (ie, numbness, dysesthesia, and paresthesia). The motor function of the head and neck is mediated through the following nerves: trigeminal (masticatory muscles), facial (muscles of expression), glossopharyngeal (uvula and soft palate), hypoglossal (tongue), and accessory (trapezius) cranial nerves.[10] Paralysis, gross weakness, atrophy, or spasticity of these muscles requires further evaluation by a neurologist.

Intraoral Evaluation

A complete dental and soft tissue examination is recommended to identify the dental, periodontal, salivary gland, or other intraoral pathoses that are suspected of causing the presenting complaints. Clinicians should be particularly aware of factors such as tongue and mucosal ridging, abnormal tooth wear, increased tooth mobility, and tenderness of the teeth to percussion that may be related to oral habits. Assess mandibular stability according to the pattern and distribution of occlusal contacts on closure. Document anterior tooth relations, including overbite and overjet, tooth-contact guidance patterns, crossbite, vertical dimension of the occlusion, and any other significant occlusal features that may be present.

Imaging

Imaging of the TMJ and craniofacial structures may be necessary to rule out structural disorders of the head, neck, and jaw. Panoramic radiographs are recommended to screen for gross tooth, periodontal, mandibular, or maxillary pathology. Special radiographic techniques such as periapical radiographs, sialography, sinus series, radionuclide studies, and angiography may be needed to rule out specific dental and other craniofacial pathology. The extensive technology available for TMJ imaging provides clinicians with multiple options.

Radiography

Radiography of the TMJ structures is prescribed primarily when clinical examination suggests some form of joint pathology.[11] Further radiographic studies should assist the diagnostic and treatment process.[12] They may include tomographic films as well as lateral pharyngeal, transorbital and modified Townes, and panoramic views of the jaws. Transcranial radiography of the TMJ joint has a limited purpose as a screening radiograph due to image distortion of the bony articular structures and superimposition of other structures.[13] Although gross degenerative or traumatic changes and the amplitude of condylar translation can be assessed by this technique, condylar position cannot[14–16]; it can be assessed only by fluoroscopy.[17]

Corrected cephalometric tomography is a more accurate method for radiographic examination of patients suspected of having articular disorders.[13,18–20] High spatial resolution of skeletal structures is obtained in multiple projections. Corrected tomography detects gross bony changes at various lateral to medial sections; thus, axially corrected tomography is preferred to transcranial projections. In normal subjects, condyle position is often centered, but considerable variability is observed. Therefore, radiographs to assess condyle position by means of joint space measurements are contraindicated for diagnostic purposes.[15,21–28] Further, condylar position in the fossa is not a diagnostic aid for articular disc displacement.[29,30]

Computerized tomography (CT) is valuable as an adjunct imaging technique for assessment of bony abnormalities of the TMJ (ie, developmental anomalies, trauma, and neoplastic conditions).[31–35] At present CT has little role in the evaluation of disc displacement because of the technical difficulty in depicting the disc.[36–38] Direct sagittal CT imaging does provide improved resolution; however, the imaging position is difficult for some patients.

In *emission scintigraphy* a radiolabeled material that is concentrated by the body in areas of rapid bone turnover is administered. A bone scan is positive if there is approximately a 10% increase in osteoblastic activity well in advance of any radiographic evidence of change. Emission imaging has high sensitivity for early stages of bony remodeling.[39,40] In *planar scintigraphy*, the area of interest is scanned with a gamma camera 2 to 4 hours after administration of the radioactive material. The areas with increased uptake of the radiolabeled material appear as "hot spots" on the scan.

Single-photon emission computed tomography (SPECT) is similar to a CT scan except that the radiation source is inside the area of interest rather than being external. While SPECT is a sensitive indicator of bone activity, it cannot discriminate between normal bone remodeling and degenerative processes. As in CT, the receptor or camera is moved about the patient, producing a tomographic slice in any plane desired. Structures under and over the plane of interest are in effect removed from the image.[41,42]

Soft Tissue Imaging

Temporomandibular joint arthrography is a radiographic technique in which radiopaque contrast medium is injected into the inferior joint space, into the superior and inferior joint spaces, or into both joint spaces followed by the introduction of air (double contrast arthrography).[43] Tomography is then used to determine the position of the articular disc relative to the condyle.[43–50] Arthrography can also reveal the functional dynamics of the disc and condyle when used with fluoroscopy and videotaping. Because of the invasiveness of the procedure, radiation, and discomfort with this imaging method, TMJ arthrography is limited to selected TMD cases of disc displacement when the dynamic imaging results will alter the course of treatment. Arthrography is the imaging study of choice for the diagnosis of disc perforation, although there is a 20% false-positive rate with the technique.[31]

Magnetic Resonance Imaging

Magnetic resonance imaging (MRI) technology is advancing at such a rapid pace that many diagnostic radiologists limit their clinical interest to this area. This imaging process is revealing pathoses and anomalous structures previously undetected and unsuspected. Magnetic resonance imaging is being increasingly utilized in the investigation of TMD.[37,51–55] Presently MRI technology affords the clinician interested in observing disc function the opportunity to view both right and left joint functions simultaneously and to interpret not only film plates but also a video that demonstrates bilaterally the symmetrical and asymmetrical excursions of the mandible, disc function, joint space, muscles of mastication, and nerve and vascular anatomy. Magnetic resonance imaging eliminates previous concern of ionizing radiation exposure and the process is painless.

The indications for MRI of the TMJ disc are the same as those for arthrography; however, increasing utilization of MRI is lessening the use of arthrography. In general, a patient should have an imaging study when the results may alter treatment strategy. This can occur when the diagnosis of articular soft tissue problems, especially in a nonreducing displaced disc with clinically restricted condylar motion, is in question or when the diagnosis must be documented for third-party payers, for medicolegal reasons, and preoperatively for disc surgery. It is important to note, however, that MRI also reveals abnormal soft tissue conditions in asymptomatic joints.[48] It has been demonstrated that between 25% and 38% of MRI of the TMJ in asymptomatic volunteers reveal disc displacement.[56–58] Thus, MRI results alone should not dictate treatment strategy.

Behavioral and Psychosocial Assessment

Basic assessment of TMD patients, especially those suffering from chronic pain, should include behavioral and psychosocial evaluation consideration. In some cases, stress-related muscle hyperactivity may be the primary contributing factor. In other cases, emotional problems such as anxiety and depression can result from unresolved signs and symptoms. Thus, it is strongly advised that the dental history include questions to evaluate behavioral, social, emotional, and cognitive factors that may initiate, sustain, or result from the patient's condition.

Comprehensive psychological inventories such as the Minnesota Multiphasic Personality Inventory (MMPI) are not necessary for routine screening.[59] The utility of most psychological tests in the dental office is limited, as the tests require interpretation in the context of an extensive psychosocial history and usually require considerable training and experience to interpret.[60] However, prior to undertaking TMD management the dentist should screen specifically for oral habits, depression, anxiety, stressful life events, lifestyle changes, secondary gain, and overuse of health care. Although in most simple cases this can be accomplished during the initial interview and examination by the dentist, further assessment is recommended if significant factors are identified. Anxiety and depression can usually be identified by simply asking the patient about these conditions.[61] Some psychological aspects of illness can be identified in TMD patients by using pain diaries or self-assessment instruments such as the Holmes and Rahe Scale for life changes.[62] Two recently developed tests, IMPATH[63] and the TMJ Scale,[64,65] are designed for use by dentists assessing TMD. A checklist of psychological and behavioral issues has recently been published and may be used by the dentist to identify factors that may warrant further evaluation from a mental health professional[66] (Fig 5-5).

If warranted, the initial psychological assessment may be followed by evaluation with a mental health care professional. In addition to the tests mentioned, the mental health care professional may use other testing instruments such as the MMPI, Hamilton Depression Scale, West Haven–Yale Multidimensional Pain Inventory, DSP & SCL-90 Scale, Beck Depression Inventory, McGill Pain Questionnaire, Multiaxial Assessment of Pain, Millon Behavioral Health Inventory, and Illness Behavior Questionnaire.[67–74] It is important to realize that these inventories should be used in the context of a careful history and clinical examination.[75]

Additional Clinical Tests

Various diagnostic studies are available for use in selected cases to assist in confirming a physical TMD diagnosis, such as biopsy, laboratory tests, and diagnostic anesthetic injections. Mounted study casts can be of value, not only as a baseline record for tooth and jaw relations, but also for evaluation of the effects of bruxism to the occlusal surface of the teeth.

Biopsy

Intra-articular biopsies are useful for benign or malignant tumors of bones, cartilage or synovium (eg, chondroma, chondrosarcoma, synovial osteochondromatosis). As previously mentioned, definitive diagnosis of temporal arteritis is usually dependent on biopsy of the temporal artery. These tests should not be considered routine procedures but rather are used to supplement knowledge gained during

---

Checklist of Psychological and Behavioral Factors

1. Inconsistent, inappropriate, and/or vague reports of pain
2. Overdramatization of symptoms
3. Symptoms that vary with life events
4. Significant pain of greater than 6 months' duration
5. Repeated failures with conventional therapies
6. Inconsistent response to medications
7. History of other stress-related disorders
8. Major life events, eg, new job, marriage, divorce, death
9. Evidence of drug abuse
10. Clinically significant anxiety or depression
11. Evidence of secondary gain

Fig 5-5 These psychosocial and behavioral considerations should be assessed as part of the patient exam and history. The significance of these factors depends on the particular patient. In general, the more factors identified, the greater is the indication that the patient should be referred to a mental health professional; however, any one of these factors may be sufficiently problematic to warrant a more extensive psychosocial evaluation.

history-taking, examination, and imaging. Soft tissue biopsy would be of primary importance for intraoral lesions and suspected neoplasia within the masticatory muscles.

Laboratory Tests

Laboratory diagnostic testing for TMD may include hematologic, urine, and synovial fluid analyses to identify hematologic, rheumatologic, metabolic, or other abnormalities suggestive of systemic disease. However, hematologic studies are rarely diagnostic of disorders that present as TMD, but they may be helpful in screening for some conditions, especially certain vascular, rheumatic, or infectious diseases. In almost all cases, a blood study that is sensitive for a particular disease is poorly specific. For example, in vascular disease like temporal arteritis, one will commonly find an elevated erythrocyte sedimentation rate (ESR), antinuclear antibodies (ANA), an anemia, and a negative rheumatoid factor (RhF). However, none of these findings alone is diagnostic. Likewise, in rheumatic disease the RhF may or may not be positive (and if positive, is not specific) and an anemia is commonly present. In the spondylarthropathies Human Lymphocyte Antigen-B27 (HLA-B27), a histocompatibility antigen, may be present in 20% to 50% of the patients but is again poorly specific for the disease.[76,77] The uric acid test is considered to be diagnostic for gouty arthritis.[78] Leucocytosis may be a sign of an acute infectious process but is again not specific for an articular infectious process. Hematologic laboratory tests that contradict the clinical diagnosis or that substantially change the intended therapy should be viewed with caution.

Analysis of synovial fluid tests for a variety of extracellular matrix (ECM) degradative enzymes, inflammatory by-products, and known pain mediators may be used as biochemical markers for the degradation that occurs with TMJ pathosis.[79–82] A study by Quinn and Bazan[83] evaluated three factors, Prostaglandin E2 (PCE2), Leukotriene B4 (LTB4), and Platelet-activating Factor (PAF) by injecting 1.5 cc of saline followed by aspiration and assay. The analysis was correlated with arthroscopic evaluation of the joint. Another study correlated keratan sulfate levels in the synovial fluid and arthroscopic examination findings.[84] There seems to be a good correlation of the degree of synovial pathosis to the level of those factors. The prime flaw in this type of research, a major drawback of any research involving invasive methods, is the lack of controls. Another use of articular fluid aspiration would be in the instance when articular infection is suspected and cultures are needed. In gout (urate crystals) and pseudogout (calcium pyrophosphate dihydrate crystals), the articular fluid can be used to analyze potential crystal formation. These two arthritides, however, are rare in the TMJ. At this point synovial fluid analysis is primarily a research tool and has little clinical application toward diagnosis and management, but future clinical value is promising because the detection of biochemical markers may precede any detection of morphologic change in the TMJ.

Diagnostic Anesthetic Injections

Diagnostic injections include neural blockade (somatic and sympathetic nerve blocks), trigger point injections, and TMJ injections. Neural blockade can be used to determine if the pain is due to pathosis peripheral to the point of the block. Lidocaine (1% to 2% without epinephrine) is recommended for diagnostic nerve blocks because it produces a prompt, longer-lasting, and more extensive anesthesia. Neural blockade is of particular prognostic value prior to neurolytic blockade or surgical sympathectomy (neurolysis). Sympathetic nerve blocks (ie, sphe-

nopalatine or stellate ganglion blocks) for diagnosis of sympathetic mediated pain should be referred to an appropriately trained anesthesiologist.[85] Myofascial trigger point injections can result in absent or decreased pain in the trigger point area and the referred pain location(s).[86] Procaine is the local anesthetic of choice for the injection of myofascial trigger points because of the low potential for adverse effects in muscles. Diagnostic anesthesia of the TMJ can be achieved by a direct lateroposterior and slightly inferior intracapsular approach to the joint, a posterior meatal intracapsular approach, or an extracapsular block of the auriculotemporal nerve at the posterior aspect of the neck of the condyle. Bupivacaine (.25%) produces prolonged anesthesia for muscle and joint diagnostic injections, but can possibly produce toxicity in muscle tissue. However, the long duration of its therapeutic effect can be very beneficial for adjunctive pain management and outweighs the reported risk of muscle toxicity.

The interpretation of diagnostic local anesthetic blocks is a challenging process requiring considerable study and caution, particularly in a patient who may have been overtreated and/or who may have developed an iatrogenic condition. Unfortunately, when well-intended treatment procedures fail, the patient's distress increases. To patients the temporary reduction in their distress (not necessarily pain relief) following an anesthetic block becomes so welcome and encouraging that they may succeed in persuading the clinician to perform an irreversible procedure. Thus, temporary relief of pain that may result following a local anesthetic block or infiltration does not always indicate that nerve ablation or surgical intervention will result in lasting relief. Diagnostic anesthetic injections are valued test procedures but they must be evaluated with the historical, clinical, and laboratory findings.

Mounted Study Casts

Articulated or mounted dental casts can facilitate detailed examination of both the static and functional relations of the teeth and jaws and serve as a baseline record for the effects of bruxism. They are of particular importance as a baseline record when orthopedic appliance therapy is contemplated because appliances can potentially cause an irreversible alteration in the tooth and jaw relations. However, acute muscle and joint pain and joint edema can decrease the accuracy of the mountings and, thus, occlusal analysis with mounted study casts is most reliable after acute disease processes are resolved.[87]

Mandibular position measurement devices that allow for the comparison of articulator condylar differences in various occlusal positions are an adjunct to mounted study casts. They provide measurements between the condylar positions in the intercuspal position and the retruded contact position in all three planes of space. Even with the most careful records and mountings, however, mounted casts are at best an approximation of the true dynamics of the mandible. The clinician should note that although mounted casts can be valuable for the study of the teeth, associated structures, and occlusal relations as an aid for dental treatment planning, they do not provide direct insight into the etiology of TMD. Thus, because the relationship between occlusion and TMD is not strongly correlated, mounted casts should not be used to diagnose TMD per se.

Proposed Additional Documentation

Numerous tests have been proposed for use in patients with TMD. Although many have potential to be clinically useful, research on their reliability and validity for TMD diagnosis has yet to be completed. All diagnostic tests should be subjected to testing for safety as well as for efficacy. Efficacy of a diagnostic test should be established through studies that determine the sensitivity, specificity, and positive and negative predictive values of the test.[88,89] The sensitivity is the probability that the test will identify disease when it is known to be present. The specificity of a test is its ability to correctly identify a patient who is free of a specific disease. The sensitivity and specificity of a test should generally be better than 70%. At this time these important characteristics are known for only a very few diagnostic tests for TMD.[90–95]

The primary concern is that with the use of many tests, a lack of scientific data can lead to many false-positive diagnoses and some false-negative diagnoses. There are immediate and implied future health and financial costs related to treating a false-positive diagnosis and the delayed costs of not treating a false-negative diagnosis. Until well-controlled clinical trials with new diagnostic tests are performed on the subgroups of TMD patients and are compared to control groups, tests should be considered experimental and should be interpreted with extreme caution.[90,92] It is hoped that as research continues a number of procedures will become accepted for specific clinical situations in the future.

Mandibular Movement Recording

Because impairment of jaw movement is one of the signs of TMD, it is not surprising that quantification of jaw movement has been considered important. Facebows using simple pens as recorders (pantography) have long been used for recording mandibular border movements lateral to the condyles. Electronic systems may enhance mandibular movement recording procedures, but their use for diagnosis depends on whether the dentist obtains diagnostically relevant information from the jaw tracking. This is an important question in view of the sparse and unreplicated scientific evidence linking jaw tracking to TMD diagnosis.[92,93,96,97] Precise tracking movements of the entire mandible in three dimensions requires a minimum of six measurements (six degrees of freedom), and the data analysis generated by such a system (especially during functional movements such as chewing) is a very complex task.[98] Instruments that measure movements at the incisors do not fulfill these requirements and are not adequate for describing molar and condylar movements or maximal mandibular movements.[99] Presently, there is insufficient scientific documentation to suggest that jaw tracking devices are useful in the diagnosis of TMD.[94] Furthermore, subjects are not able to consistently reproduce functional jaw movements even after training.[100,101]

Electromyography

Electromyography (EMG) can be useful for studies of reflex activity and nerve conduction and for the assessment of parafunctional behavior. Parafunctional activity can be monitored and in some instances can be recorded outside of the dental office by means of diurnal or nocturnal electronic measuring techniques. The measurement of other functional and postural acts by surface EMG is less useful because variations in means exceed the very differences one seeks to establish between "normal" and "abnormal" subject groups.[92,102–104] A recent comprehensive review of the scientific literature[94] concluded that there is not yet sufficient evidence to support the use of EMG for

the evaluation or diagnosis of TMD. This is consistent with conclusions reached during scientific conferences of the Neuroscience Group of the International Association for Dental Research,[105] a workshop of the National Institute of Dental Research (NIH, April 3 to 4, 1989), and scientific programs dealing with diagnosis of TMD by the American Academy of Craniomandibular Disorders (Washington, DC, April 13 to 15, 1989) and the European Academy of Craniomandibular Disorders (Zürich, Switzerland, October 8 to 10, 1987).

Thermography

The diagnosis of neurologic and musculoskeletal abnormalities by thermography is based on thermal asymmetry between normal and abnormal sites. The applicability of thermography to the diagnosis of TMD has been addressed with conflicting results.[106,107] The concept is that if normal pain-free subjects have symmetrical thermograms,[108] then asymmetrical thermograms might suggest the presence of TMD. Some studies indicate that TMD patients have increased thermal emission on the symptomatic side,[109,110] especially the affected joint.[111] However, a study by Finney et al[112] suggests that TMD patients have decreased thermal emission on the symptomatic side. The variability of normal facial surface temperature between sides may be considerable.[113] A recent comprehensive review found that there is conflicting evidence on the direction of temperature shift over the painful site and high within-patient and between-patient variability.[95] Studies demonstrate that the results of thermography can vary greatly according to technique and instrument position. The results of clinical investigations suggest that thermographic "hot spots" in the back are unassociated with active trigger points and "cold patches" on the face or head are not prognostic for headache.[114,115] Presently, there is little scientific evidence to suggest that thermography is useful in the diagnosis of TMD.[116,117]

Mediate Auscultation

Sonography is the technique of recording and graphically representing sound. In Doppler ultrasonography (the application of the Doppler effect to ultrasonic scanning), ultrasound echoes are converted to amplified audible sound waves as the ultrasonic transmissions bounce off moving tissues within the TMJ. The clinical significance and reproducibility of sounds emanating from the TMJ are still not clear.[101,118] One study compared clinical findings and arthrographic data to Doppler ultrasonographic findings.[119] Although this and other longitudinal data are available,[120,121] more information is needed before the clinical significance of these sounds can be better understood.[122] Recent comprehensive reviews concluded that there is no clinical advantage of using sonography or Doppler methods over a conventional stethoscope or direct auscultation to document joint sounds.[92,94,123]

References

1. Dworkin SF, Le Resche L, De Rouen T, Von Korff M: Assessing clinical signs of temporomandibular disorders: Reliability of clinical examiners. J Prosthet Dent 1990;63:574–579.

2. Griffith RH: Report of the President's Conference of the Examination, Diagnosis, and Management of Temporomandibular Disorders. J Am Dent Assoc 1983; 106:75–78.

3. Clark GT, Seligman DA, Solberg WK, Pullinger AG: Guidelines for the examination and diagnosis of temporomandibular disorders. J Craniomandib Disord Facial Oral Pain 1989;3:7–14.

4. Schiffman E, Fricton J, Haley D, Tylka D: A pressure algometer for myofascial pain syndrome: Reliability and validity testing. In Dubner R, et al (eds) Proceedings of the Fifth World Congress on Pain. Vol 3. Amsterdam, Elsevier, 1988, pp 407–413.

5. Ohrbach R, Gale EN: Pressure pain thresholds, clinical assessment, and differential diagnosis: reliability and validity in patients with myogenic pain. Pain 1989; 39:157–169.

6. List T, Helkimo M, Karlsson R: Influence of pressure rates on the reliability of a pressure threshold meter. J Craniomandib Disord Facial Oral Pain 1991;5:173–178.

7. Clark GT: Examining temporomandibular disorder patients for craniocervical dysfunction. J Craniomand Pract 1984; 2:56–63.

8. Clark GT, Green EM, Dornan MR, Flack VF: Craniocervical dysfunction levels in a patient sample from a temporomandibular joint clinic. J Am Dent Assoc 1987; 115:251–256.

9. Sjaastad O, Fredriksen TA, Pfaffenrath V: Cervicogenic headache: Diagnostic criteria. Headache 1990;30:725–726.

10. Tanaka, TT: Recognition of the pain formula for head, neck, and TMJ disorders. V: The general physical examination. J Calif Dent Assoc 1984;12:43–49.

11. Lindvall AM, Helkimo E, Hollender L, Carlsson GE: Radiographic examination fo the temporomandibular joint. A comparison between radiographic findings and gross and microscopic morphologic observations. Dentomaxillofac Radiol 1976; 5:24–32.

12. Hatcher DC: Craniofacial imaging. J Calif Dent Assoc 1991;19:27–34.

13. Knoernschild KL, Aquilino SA, Ruprecht A: Transcranial radiography and linear

tomography: A comparative study. J Prosthet Dent 1991;66:239–250.

14. Oberg T, Carlsson GE, Fajers CM: The temporomandibular joint. A morphologic study on a human autopsy material. Acta Odontol Scand 1971;29:349–384.

15. Dixon DC, Graham GS, Mayhew RB, Oesterle LJ, Simms D, Pierson WP: The validity of transcranial radiography in diagnosing TMJ anterior disk displacement. J Am Dent Assoc 1984;108:615–618.

16. Aquilino SA, Matteson SR, Holland GA, Phillips C: Evaluation of condylar position from temporomandibular joint radiographs. J Prosthet Dent 1985;53:88–97.

17. Preti G, Fava C: Lateral transcranial radiography of temporomandibular joints. Part I: Validity in skulls and patients. J Prosthet Dent 1988;59:85–93.

18. Hansson LG, Hansson T, Petersson A: A comparison between clinical and radiologic findings in 259 temporomandibular joint patients. J Prosthet Dent 1983;50:89–94.

19. Petersson A, Rohlin M: Rheumatoid arthritis of the temporomandibular joint. Evaluation of three different radiographic techniques by assessment of observer performance. Dentomaxillofac Radiol 1988;17:115–120.

20. Ludlow JB, Nolan PJ, McNamara JA: Accuracy of measures of the temporomandibular joint space and condylar position with three tomographic imaging techniques. Oral Surg Oral Med Oral Pathol 1991;72:364–370.

21. Blaschke DD, Blaschke TJ: Normal TMJ bony relationships in centric occlusion. J Dent Res 1981;60:98–104.

22. American Dental Association: Recommendations in radiographic practices, 1984 Council on Dental Materials, Instruments, and Equipment. J Am Dent Assoc 1984;109:764–765.

23. Pullinger AG, Hollender L, Solberg WK, Petersson A: A tomographic study of mandibular condyle position in an asymptomatic population. J Prosthet Dent 1985;53:706–713.

24. Pullinger AG, Solberg WK, Hollender L, Guichet D: Tomographic analysis of mandibular condyle position in diagnostic subgroups of temporomandibular disorders. J Prosthet Dent 1986;55:723–729.

25. Rohlin M, Akerman S, Kopp S: Tomography as an aid to detect macroscopic changes of the TMJ. An autopsy study of the aged. Acta Odont Scand 1986;44:131–140.

26. Ronquillo HI, Guay J, Tallents RH, Katzberg RW, Murphy W: Tomographic analysis of mandibular condyle position compared to arthrographic findings of the TMJ. J Craniomandib Disord Facial Oral Pain 1988;2:59–64.

27. Herbosa EG, Rotskoff KS, Ramos FB, Ambrookian HS: Condylar position in superior maxillary repositioning and its effect on the temporomandibular joint. J Oral Maxillofac Surg 1990;48:690–696.

28. Pandis N, Karpac J, Trevino R, Williams B: A radiographic study of condyle position at various depths of cut in dry skulls with axially corrected lateral tomograms. Am J Orthod Dentofac Orthop 1991;100:116–122.

29. Katzberg RW, Keith DA, Ten Eick WR, Guralnick WC: Internal derangements of the TMJ: An assessment of condylar position with centric occlusion. J Prosthet Dent 1983;49:250–254.

30. Brand JW, Whitnery JG, Anderson ON, Keenan KM: Condylar position as a predictor of temporomandibular joint internal derangement. Oral Surg 1989;67:469–476.

31. Helms CA, Morrish RB, Kircos LT, Katzberg RW, Dolwick WF: Computed tomography of the meniscus of the temporomandibular joint: Preliminary observations. Radiology 1982;145:719–722.

32. Manzione JV, Katzberg RW, Brodsky GL, Seltzer SE, Mellins HZ: Internal derangements of the temporomandibular joint:

Diagnosis by direct sagittal computed tomography. Radiology 1984;150:111–115.

33. Manco LG, Messing SG, Busino LJ, Fasulo CP, Sordill WC: Internal derangements of the temporomandibular joint evaluated with direct sagittal CT. Radiology 1985;157:407–412.

34. Raustia AM, Phytinen J, Virtanen KK: Examination of the temporomandibular joint by direct sagittal computed tomography. Clin Radiol 1985;36:291–296.

35. Paz ME, Katzberg RW, Tallents RH, Westesson P-L, Proskin HM, Murphy WC: CT evaluation of the TMJ disk. Oral Surg Oral Med Oral Pathol 1988;66:519–524.

36. Christiansen EL, Thompson JR, Hasso AN, Hinshaw DB, Moore RJ, Roberts D, Kopp S: CT number characteristics of malpositioned TMJ menisci. Diagnosis with CT number highlighting (blink mode). Invest Radiol 1987;22:315–321.

37. Westesson PL, Katzberg RW, Tallents RH, Woodworth RE, Svensson SA: CT & MR of the TMJ: Comparison with autopsy specimens. Am J Roentgenol 1987; 148:1165–1171.

38. Fava C, Gatti G, Cardes E, Parchetti R, Rocca G, Preti G: Possibilities and limits in identifying the TMJ articular meniscus with the CT scanner: A comparative anatomoradiological study. J Craniomandib Disord Facial Oral Pain 1988;2:141–147.

39. Goldstein HA, Bloom CY: Detection of degenerative disease of the temporomandibular joint by bone scintigraphy: Concise communication. J Nucl Med 1980; 21:928–930.

40. Kircos, LT, Ortendahl DA, Hattner RS, Faulkner D, Chafetz NI, Taylor RC: Emission imaging of patients with craniomandibular dysfunction. Oral Surg Oral Med Oral Pathol 1988;65:249–254.

41. Katzberg RW, O'Mara RE, Tallents RH, Weber DA: Radionuclide skeletal imaging and SPECT in suspected internal derangements of the TMJ. J Oral Maxillofac Surg 1984;42:782–787.

42. Krasnow AZ, Collier BD, Kneeland JB, et al: Comparison of high-resolution MRI and SPECT bone scintigraphy for noninvasive imaging of the TMJ. J Nucl Med 1987;28:1268–1274.

43. Westesson PL, Bronstein DI: Temporomandibular joint: Comparison of single and double-contrast arthrography. Radiology 1985;164:65–70.

44. Katzberg RW, Dolwick MF, Helms CA, Hopens T, Bales DJ, Coggs GC: Arthrotomography of the temporomandibular joint. Am J Roentgenol 1980;134:995–1003.

45. Westesson PL: Double-contrast arthrography of the TMJ: Introduction of a technique. J Oral Maxillofac Surg 1983; 41:163–172.

46. Roberts CA, Tallents RA, Espeland MA, Handelman SL, Katzberg RW: Mandibular range of motion versus arthrographic diagnosis of the TMJ. Oral Surg Oral Med Oral Pathol 1985;60:244–251.

47. Roberts CA, Katzberg RW, Tallents RA, Espeland MA, Handelman SL: Correlation of clinical parameters to the arthrographic depiction of TMJ internal derangements. Oral Surg Oral Med Oral Pathol 1988;66:32–36.

48. Kozeniauskas JJ, Ralph WJ: Bilateral arthrographic evaluation of unilateral TMJ pain and dysfunction. J Prosthet Dent 1988;60:98–105.

49. Liedberg L, Westesson PL: Sideways position of the TMJ disk: Coronal cryosectioning of fresh autopsy specimens. Oral Surg Oral Med Oral Pathol 1988;66:644–649.

50. Rohrer FA, Palla S, Engelke W: Condylar movements including joints before and after arthrography. J Oral Rehabil 1991; 18:111–123.

51. Carr AB, Gibilisco JA, Berquist TH: Magnetic resonance imaging of the temporomandibular joint—preliminary work. J Craniomandib Disord Oral Facial Pain 1987;1:89–96.

52. Donlon WC, Moon KL: Comparison of magnetic resonance imaging, arthrotomography and clinical and surgical findings in temporomandibular joint internal derangements. Oral Surg Oral Med Oral Pathol 1987;64:2–5.

53. Sanchez-Woodworth RE, Tallents RH, Katzberg RW, Guay JA: Bilateral internal derangements of the TMJ: Evaluation by MRI imaging. Oral Surg Oral Med Oral Pathol 1988;65:281–285.

54. Helms CA, Kaban LB, McNeill C, Dodson T: Temporomandibular joint: Morphology and signal intensity characteristics of the disc at MR imaging. Radiology 1989;172:817–820.

55. Helms CA, Doyle GW, Orwig D, McNeill C, Kaban L: Staging of internal derangements of the TMJ with magnetic resonance imaging: Preliminary observations. J Craniomandib Disord Facial Oral Pain 1989;3:93–99.

56. Moore JB, et al: Coronal and sagittal TMJ meniscus position in asymptomatic subjects by MRI. J Oral Maxillofac Surg 1989;47 (suppl 1):75.

57. Kircos LT, Ortendahl DA, Mark AS, et al: Magnetic resonance imaging of the TMJ disc in asymptomatic volunteers. J Oral Maxillofac Surg 1987;45:397–401.

58. Hatala MP, Westesson P-L, Tallents RH, Katzberg RW: TMJ disc displacement in asymptomatic volunteers as detected by MR imaging. J Dent Res 1991 (special issue);70:27, abstr 100.

59. Olson RE: Behavioral Examinations in MPD. In Laskin DM, Greenfield W, Gale E, Rugh J, Neff P, Alling C, Ayer WA (eds) The President's Conference on the Examination, Diagnosis, and Management of Temporomandibular Disorders. Chicago, American Dental Association, 1983, pp 104–105.

60. Harness DM, Rome HP: Psychological and behavior aspects of chronic facial pain. Otolaryngol Clin North Am 1989;22:1073–1074.

61. Gale EN, Dixon DC: A simplified psychologic questionnaire as a treatment planning aid for patients with temporomandibular disorders. J Prosthet Dent 1989;61:235–238.

62. Moody PM, Kemper JT, Okeson JP, Calhoun TC, Packer MV: Recent life changes and myofascial pain syndrome. J Prosthet Dent 1982;48:328–330.

63. Fricton JR, Nelson A, Monsein M: Impath: Microcomputer assessment of behavioral and psychological factors in craniomandibular disorders. J Craniomand Pract 1987;5:372–381.

64. Levitt SR, McKinney MW, Lundeen TF. The TMJ scale: Cross-variation and reliability studies. J Craniomand Pract 1988;6:18–25.

65. Lundeen TF, Levitt SR, McKinney MW: Clinical applications of the TMJ Scale. J Craniomand Pract 1988;6:339–345.

66. McNeill C, Mohl ND, Rugh JD, Tanaka TT: Temporomandibular disorders: Diagnosis, management, education, and research. J Am Dent Assoc 1990;120:253–260.

67. Beck AT, Ward CH, Mendelson M, Mock J, Erbaugh J: An inventory for measuring depression. Arch Gen Psychiat 1961;4:564–571.

68. Melzack R: The McGill pain questionnaire: Major properties and scoring methods. Pain 1975;1:277–299.

69. Millon T, Green C, Meagher R: Millon Behavioral Health Inventory Manual. Minneapolis, National Computer Systems, 1982.

70. Speculand B, Goss AN: Psychological factors in temporomandibular joint dysfunction pain. Int J Oral Surg 1985;14:131–137.

71. Eversole LR, Machado L: Temporomandibular joint internal derangements and associated neuromuscular disorders. J Am Dent Assoc 1985;110:69–79.

72. Kerns RD, Turk DC, Rudy TE: The West Haven-Yale multidimensional pain inventory (WHYMPI). Pain 1985;23:345–386.

73. Gerschman JA, Wright JL, Hall WD,

Reade PC, Burrows GD, Howell BJ: Comparisons of psychological and social factors in patients with chronic oro-facial pain and dental phobic disorders. Aust Dent J 1987;32:222–225.

74. Turk DC, Rudy TE: Towards a comprehensive assessment of chronic pain patients. Behav Res Ther 1987;25:237–249.

75. Rugh JD: Validity of psychological testing in TMD. In McNeill C (ed) Current Controversies in Temporomandibular Disorders. Chicago, Quintessence Publ Co, 1992, pp 138–142.

76. Beary JF, Christian CL, Sculco TP (eds): Manual of Rheumatology and Outpatient Orthopedic Disorders. Boston, Little, Brown & Co, 1982, pp 44–185.

77. Wyngaarden JB, Smith LH: Cecil Textbook of Medicine. Vols I, II. Philadelphia, WB Saunders Co, 1985, pp 1932, 1891–1895.

78. German DC, Holmes EW: Hypo-uricemia and gout. Med Clin North Am 1986; 70:419–436.

79. Fujiwara Y: Paper-electrophoretic study of proteins. Glycoproteins and lipoproteins in human synovial fluid. J Jpn Orthop Assoc 1964;38:339–863.

80. Kakudo K, Takasu J, Yamamoto S: Ultrastructural observations of horseradish peroxidase in synovial lining cells of the rats' temporomandibular joint. J Dent Res 1977;56:1376.

81. Kakudo K: Ultrastructural cytochemical studies of horseradish peroxidase uptake by synovial lining cells of the rat temporomandibular joint. Okajima Folia Anat Jpn 1980;57:219–240.

82. Kubo Y: The uptake of horseradish peroxidase in monkey temporomandibular joint synovium after occlusal alteration. J Dent Res 1987;66:1049–1054.

83. Quinn JH, Bazan NG: Identification of prostaglandin E2 and leukotriene B4 in the synovial fluid of painful, dysfunctional temporomandibular joints. J Oral Maxillofac Surg 1990;48:968–971.

84. Israel HA, Saed-Nejad F, Ratcliffe A: Early diagnosis of osteoarthrosis of temporomandibular joint: Correlation between arthroscopic diagnosis and keratan sulfate levels in the synovial fluid. J Oral Maxillofac Surg 1991;49:708–711.

85. Waldman SD: The role of neural blockade in the evaluation and treatment of common headache and facial pain syndromes. Headache Q 1991;2:286–291.

86. Travell JG, Simons DG: Myofascial Pain and Dysfunction: The Trigger Point Manual. Baltimore, Williams and Wilkins, 1983, pp 63–158.

87. Dyer EH: Importance of a stable maxillomandibular relation. J Prosthet Dent 1973;30:241–242.

88. Douglass CW, McNeill BJ: Clinical decision analysis methods applied to diagnostic tests in dentistry. J Dent Educ 1983; 47:709–712.

89. Mohl ND: Temporomandibular disorders: The role of occlusion, TMJ imaging, and electronic devices. J Am College Dent 1991;58:4–10.

90. Greene CS: Can technology enhance TM disorder diagnosis? J Calif Dent Assoc 1990;18:21–24.

91. Goulet J-P, Clark GT: Clinical TMJ examination methods. J Calif Dent Assoc 1990;18:25–33.

92. Widmer CG, Lund JP, Feine JS: Evaluation of diagnostic tests for TMD. J Calif Dent Assoc 1990;18:53–60.

93. Mohl ND, McCall WS, Lund JP, Plesh O: Devices for the diagnosis and treatment of temporomandibular disorders: Part I. Introduction, scientific evidence, and jaw tracking. J Prosthet Dent 1990;63:198–201.

94. Mohl ND, Lund JP, Widmer CG, McCall WD: Devices for the diagnosis and treatment of temporomandibular disorders. Part II. Electromyography and sonography. J Prosthet Dent 1990;63:332–336.

95. Mohl ND, Ohrbach RK, Crow HC, Gross AJ: Devices for the diagnosis and treatment of temporomandibular disorders. Part III. Thermography, ultrasound, elec-

trical stimulation and EMG biofeedback. J Prosthet Dent 1990c;63:472–477.

96. Feine JS, Hutchins MD, Lund JP: An evaluation of the criteria used to diagnose mandibular dysfunction with the mandibular kinesiograph. J Prosthet Dent 1988; 60:374–380.

97. Velasco J, Tasaki T, Gale E: Study of pantographic tracings of TMD patients and asymptomatic subjects. J Dent Res 1991;70(special issue):abstr 843.

98. Gibbs C, Lundeen H: Jaw movements and forces during chewing and swallowing and their clinical significance. In Lundeen H, Gibbs C (eds) Advances in Occlusion. Boston, John Wright, 1982, pp 2–32.

99. Balkhi KM, Tallents RH, Goldin B, Catania JA: Error analysis of a magnetic jaw-tracking device. J Craniomandib Disord Facial Oral Pain 1991;5:51–56.

100. dos Santos J Jr, Ash MM Jr, Warshawsky P: Learning to reproduce consistent functional jaw movement. J Prosthet Dent 1991;65:294–302.

101. Toolsen GA, Sadowsky C: An evaluation of the relationship between temporomandibular joint sounds and mandibular movement. J Craniomandib Disord Facial Oral Pain 1991;5:187–196.

102. Lund JP, Widmer CG: Evaluation of the use of surface electromyography in the diagnosis, documentation and treatment of dental patients. J Craniomandib Disord Facial Oral Pain 1989;3:125–137.

103. Rugh JD, Davis SE: Accuracy of diagnosing MPD using electromyography. J Dent Res 1990;69(special issue):273, abstr 1319.

104. Schroeder H, Siegmund H, Santibanez H-G, Kluge A: Causes and signs of temporomandibular joint pain and dysfunction: An electromyographical investigation. J Oral Rehabil 1991;18:301–310.

105. International Association of Dental Research. Newsletter. Vol 3, No. 6, 1987.

106. Pogrel MA, Yen CK, Taylor RC: Infrared thermography in oral and maxillofacial surgery. Oral Surg Oral Med Oral Pathol 1989;67:126–131.

107. Pogrel MA, Erbez G, Taylor RC, Dodson TB: Liquid crystal thermography as a diagnostic aid and objective monitor for TMJ dysfunction and myogenic facial pain. J Craniomand Disord Facial Oral Pain 1989;3:65–70.

108. Feldman F, Nickoloff EL: Normal thermographic standards for the cervical spine and upper extremities. Skeletal Radiol 1984;12:235–349.

109. Berry DC, Yemm R: Variations in skin temperature on the face in normal subjects and in patients with mandibular dysfunction. Br J Oral Surg 1971;8:242–247.

110. Berry DC, Yemm R: A further study of facial skin temperature in patients with mandibular dysfunction. J Oral Rehabil 1974;1:255–264.

111. Steed PA: The utilization of contact liquid crystal thermography in the evaluation of temporomandibular dysfunction. J Craniomand Pract 1991;9:120–128.

112. Finney JW, Holt CR, Pearce KB: Thermographic diagnosis of temporomandibular joint disease and associated neuromuscular disorders. Postgrad Med Special Rep, Proceedings of the Academy of Neuromuscular Thermography. March, 1986, pp 93–95.

113. Johansson A, Kopp S, Haraldson T: Reproducibility and variation of skin surface temperature over the temporomandibular joint and masseter muscle in normal individuals. Acta Odontol Scand 1985;43:309–313.

114. Swerdlow B, Dieter JN: The vascular "cold patch" is not a prognostic index for headache. Headache 1989;29:562–568.

115. Swerdlow B, Dieter JN: An evaluation of the sensitivity and specificity of medical thermography for the documentation of myofascial trigger points. Pain 1992;48:205–213.

116. Gratt BM, Pullinger A, Sickles EA, Lee JJ: Electronic thermography of normal facial structures: A pilot study. Oral Surg Oral Med Oral Pathol 1989a;68:346–351.

117. Gratt BM, Sickles EA, Graff-Radford SB, Solberg W: Electronic thermography in the diagnosis of atypical odontalgia: A pilot study. Oral Surg Oral Med Oral Pathol 1989b;68:472–481.

118. Hardeson JD, Okeson JP: Comparison of three clinical techniques for evaluating joint sounds. J Craniomand Pract 1990;8:307–311.

119. Davidson SL: Doppler auscultation. J Craniomandib Disord Facial Oral Pain 1988;2:128–132.

120. Gay T, Bertolamie CN: Arthrophonometry of the TMJ. J Dent Res 1986;65(special issue):abstr 851.

121. Heffez L, Blaustein D: Advances in sonography of the temporomandibular joint. Oral Surg Oral Med Oral Pathol 1986;62:486–495.

122. Greene CS, Laskin DM: Long term status of TMJ clicking in patients with myofascial pain dysfunction. J Am Dent Assoc 1988;117:461–465.

123. Widmer CG: Temporomandibular joint sounds: A critique of techniques for recording and analysis. J Craniomandib Disord Facial Oral Pain 1989;3:213–217.

Management

Management goals for patients with TMD are similar to those for patients with other orthopedic or rheumatologic disorders, namely, decreased pain, decreased adverse loading, restored function, and restored normal daily activities. These goals are best achieved by a well-defined program designed to treat the physical and/or psychological disorder(s) and to decrease or remove all contributing factors. The management options and sequence of treatments for TMD described here are consistent with treatment of other musculoskeletal disorders.

As in many musculoskeletal conditions, the signs and symptoms of TMD may be transient and self-limiting, resolving without serious long-term effects.[1-3] Little is known about which signs and symptoms will progress to more serious conditions in the natural course of TMD. For these reasons, a special effort should be made to avoid aggressive, nonreversible therapy, such as complex occlusal therapy or surgery. Conservative treatment such as behavioral modification, physical therapy, medications, and orthopedic appliances are endorsed for the initial care of nearly all TMD.[4]

The majority of patients suffering with TMD achieve good relief of symptoms with conservative therapy.[5,6] Long-term follow-up of TMD patients shows that more than 50% of the patients have few or no symptoms after conservative treatment. From a study of 154 patients, it was concluded that most TMD patients have minimal recurrent symptoms 7 years after conservative treatment procedures.[2] A study of 90 patients with clinically documented TMD who were followed for 10 years revealed that more than 90% had relief of symptoms after conservative treatment.[7] In a recent study of 110 TMD patients, 85.5% reported that they experienced no pain or much less pain at 2.0 to 8.5 years after conservative treatment.[8] In many patients with disc displacement, painless and satisfactory function are possible although the disc remains displaced.[9] In fact, patients with disc displacement of the temporomandibular joint may go through a natural progression of healing and remodeling.[10,11]

It is strongly suggested that the use of the terms phase I and phase II treatment of TMD be discontinued. Phase I therapy usually referred to behavior modification, counseling, pharmacotherapy, physical therapy, and/or orthopedic appliances. In the past, phase II therapy traditionally referred to some form of definitive occlusal therapy, ie, equilibration, restorative therapy, full-mouth reconstruction, prosthodontic therapy, orthodontic therapy and/or orthognathic surgery, or surgery. The disturbing concern with phase I/phase II terminology is that to some, if not to many, dentists the concept of two phases of treatment means that after completing phase I treatment, phase II treatment is automatically planned. But the scientific literature does not support the need for a two-phase approach because definitive occlusal therapy is not required for most TMD cases. The need for follow-up or second-phase occlusal therapy is a historical belief system that dentists have developed, in part, from previous predoctoral and postdoctoral programs, and, in the main, from continuing education courses. Although the literature does not support a direct correlation between occlusion and TMD, and thus the need for phase II TMD therapy, it does not exclude occlusal therapy as valid for the proper treatment of numerous dental conditions.

Despite the success of conservative care, some patients with TMD do not improve. Reasons for this vary but these patients generally fall into two groups: (1) patients with pain and dysfunction caused by major structural changes in the joint, and (2) patients with a chronic pain syndrome complicated by multiple contributing factors. In the first situation, TMJ surgery may be indicated. In the second situation, a chronic pain management program with a team of clinicians may be needed. A treatment team is needed because it is difficult for an individual clinician to address the multitude of contributing factors that may be present in complex chronic pain patients.[12]

Traditionally, most treatment of TMD has been unique and varied according to the clinician's favorite theory of causation.[6] As a result, success of treatment was often compromised by limited approaches that only addressed part of the problem. With a team, various aspects of the problem can be addressed by different specialists, which enhances the overall potential for success. Teams can be interdisciplinary (one setting) or multidisciplinary (multiple settings). Management goals are best achieved by using the optimal combination and sequence of treatment options in the context of the overall management program. All management programs should be time limited. Treatment options include (1) patient education and self-care, (2) cognitive intervention, (3) psychotherapy, (4) pharmacotherapy, (5) physical therapy, (6) orthopedic appliance therapy, (7) occlusal therapy, and (8) surgery. Each of these modalities will be discussed in detail separately, but in practice they should be used in combination depending on the needs of the patient.

Patient Education and Self-Care

The success of a self-care program depends on patient motivation, cooperation, and compliance. The clinician must take the time to explain the clinical findings, diagnostic data, treatment options, and prognosis to the patient. The time spent on patient reassurance and education is a significant factor in developing a high level of rapport and treatment compliance. This requires attentive listening on the part of the clinician and sufficient time for the patient to present his concerns. A careful explanation of the problem and treatment plan, using terminology the patient can understand, is important to successful management.

A successful self-care program may allow healing and prevent further injury to the musculoskeletal system and is often enough to control the problem.[6,13] Instruction in a self-care routine should include the following: rest of the musculoskeletal system through voluntary limitation of mandibular function, habit awareness and modification, and a home physiotherapeutic program. An explanation of the advantages of resting the affected muscular and articular structures, much the same as an athlete must rest or immobilize an injured joint, is most helpful. This explanation should emphasize function modification (ie, avoidance of heavy mastication, gum chewing, wide yawning, singing) and habit awareness (ie, avoidance of clenching, bruxing, tongue thrusting, poor sleeping posture, object biting, and playing certain musical instruments).[14] Habit change can be accomplished when the patient becomes more aware of the habit, knows how to correct it, and has the motivation to correct it. When this knowledge is combined with a commitment to conscientious monitoring, some habits will change. A simple form of feedback, such as visual reminders adapted to the patient's daily activities, should be discussed and implemented (eg, small stickers strategically placed at home, in the automobile, and at work). The feedback objects should remind the patient to be aware of the habit and then to help modify it. Progress with habit modification should be addressed at all appointments with the patient.

A home physiotherapeutic program is also beneficial.[15] When such a program is

described in detail, further enhancement of the doctor-patient relationship and compliance results. Emphasis on patient self-control should remain a paramount theme. A program of moist heat or ice or both to the affected areas, massage of the affected muscles, and gentle range of motion exercises can decrease tenderness and pain and increase range of motion. Heat is commonly applied with hot compresses, moist heating pads, hydrocollators, and disposable hot packs. These applications transmit heat by conduction and are only useful for superficial heating (1 to 5 mm in depth). Heat stimulates analgesia, muscle relaxation, and improvement in the physiologic state of the tissue. Cold, used primarily for its local analgesic and anti-inflammatory effects in muscle tissue, is applied to the affected area by ice that is moved along the direction of the muscle fibers for several minutes. Because cold is uncomfortable, however, it is best to warm the area afterward. Alternate application of heat, ice, and heat again may be most effective. Because the temperature differential is greater with cold, a shorter application may produce a greater response. Heat should not be used for acute injury (less than 72 hours), acute inflammation, or infection. Cold should not be used over areas with poor circulation (as found in patients with diabetes) or over open wounds.

Cognitive Behavioral Intervention

Approaches to changing maladaptive habits and behavior is an important part of the overall treatment program for TMD patients.[16] Although simple habits may be modified when the patient is made aware of them, changing persistent habits may require a structured program that is facilitated by a clinician trained in behavioral modification.[17-19] Significant modification in the patient's lifestyle is often necessary to alter the contributing factors. If a more structured approach is indicated, strategies for behavior modification such as a habit reversal program, lifestyle counseling, progressive relaxation, hypnosis, and biofeedback should be considered. Treatment should be individualized to best fit the patient's problems, preferences, and lifestyle.

Biofeedback is a structured therapy based on the theory that when an individual receives information about a desired change and is supported for making the change, the change is more likely to occur.[20] In general, biofeedback training uses equipment to measure biological activity (eg, surface electromyograph to measure muscle activity). The equipment is designed with a "feedback" loop so that a patient can receive immediate information (feedback). A number of controlled studies have demonstrated that relaxation training, with or without the use of surface electromyographic (EMG) biofeedback, can decrease diurnal (daytime) tonic muscle activity.[18] The use of nocturnal EMG biofeedback has been reported to be effective in controlling nighttime bruxism.[21-23] However, such studies have generally been of short duration, and the short-term biofeedback therapy has not been followed by measurable long-term decreases in bruxing behavior.[24,25] Because nocturnal EMG biofeedback without a more comprehensive stress management program appears to decrease bruxism only temporarily, its use may be limited to short-term management of acute conditions.

Comprehensive stress management and counseling programs that involve a combination of EMG biofeedback, progressive relaxation, and self-directed changes in lifestyle appear to be more effective than is any single behavioral treatment procedure. Use of behavioral therapies in conjunction with dental therapies appears to enhance the overall therapeutic effects.[26]

Psychotherapy

The plethora of emotional and interpersonal connotations associated with the functions of the mouth and jaw make these anatomic sites the ideal focus for the symbolic portrayal of psychological conflicts.[27,28] For some TMD patients, symptoms may serve as a somatic metaphor that both expresses and resolves pre-existing or concurrent psychological conflicts.[29,30] Chronic pain behaviors may both enact and inhibit aggressive, dependent, and sexual impulses that the patient both wishes and fears.[31,32] Thus, symptoms may be a compromise formation that decreases anxiety and conflict while facilitating the patient's unconscious, involuntary best effort to function adaptively.[33] These primary gains of symptom formation may be offset by the limitations and discomfort that accompany TMD and orofacial pain conditions.

When TMD and orofacial pain are symptoms of a true conversion disorder or are integrally part of the patient's characterologic defensive and coping style, treatment efforts with pharmacologic or cognitive-behavioral management alone are likely to prove insufficient.[29] These patients should be referred to a mental health professional skilled in gaining access to and resolving psychological conflicts. The goal of psychotherapeutic intervention is to translate the meaning of the somatic symptom into its psychological and interpersonal equivalents, and then to help the patient resolve the original conflicts. These efforts often extend beyond the resolution of the original TMD or orofacial pain symptoms.[34–36] The role of the dentist is to insure continuity of treatment by providing supportive involvement and routine dental care. At the same time, invasive or irreversible dental procedures are to be assiduously avoided.[37] Careful coordination of treatment by the dentist and mental health professional will assure that such patients receive optimal care.[38,39]

Pharmacotherapy

Both clinical experience and controlled experimental studies show that pharmacotherapy can be a powerful catalyst to patient comfort and rehabilitation when used as part of a comprehensive management program.[40] Although there is a tendency for clinicians to rely on a single "favorite" agent, no one drug has a proven efficacy for the entire spectrum of TMD. To avoid unexpected complications and adverse drug interactions and to achieve maximal efficacy, it is important to become familiar with a spectrum of drugs that may be prescribed for orofacial pain.

Of concern with TMD pharmacotherapy are the problems that can occur with drug misuse or abuse. Because opioid narcotics produce tolerance and dependence, continued analgesic usage in the TMD patient needs careful consideration.[41–43] The use of "prn" (as needed) pain-contingent drug prescribing is still common despite clear warnings in the literature that this approach is ineffective and may lead to abuse with some patients. Therefore, dependence-producing pharmaceuticals should only be used on a time-contingent basis.[44] Every other avenue of treatment should be pursued rather than relying on narcotic medication for TMD patients.

For patients with chronic orofacial pain including TMD pain, the risks of psycho-tropic medications, including the benzodiazepines (eg, central nervous system [CNS] depression), are likely to outweigh the therapeutic benefits. Rarely indicated for specific TMD, anticonvulsant medications may be prescribed by appropriately trained clinicians for diagnostic and therapeutic reasons for orofacial pain syndromes of neuropathic origin; however, careful monitoring is essential for patient safety. For proper management of TMD patients with chronic pain secondary to pre-existing or concurrent psychiatric disorders, psychoactive medications should be prescribed by a psychiatrist in conjunction with comprehensive care for the patient's overall mental health needs.

The most effective pharmacologic agents for the management of TMD include analgesics, nonsteroidal anti-inflammatory drugs (NSAID), corticosteroids, muscle relaxants, and antidepressants.[45–47] The analgesics and corticosteroids are indicated for acute TMD pain, the nonsteroidal anti-inflammatory agents and muscle relaxants may be used for both acute and chronic conditions, and the tricyclic antidepressants are primarily indicated for chronic orofacial pain management.[48,49]

Analgesics

Analgesics, either opiate or nonopiate preparations, are used to reduce pain associated with TMD. The nonopiate analgesics are a heterogeneous group of compounds that share certain therapeutic actions and side effects.[50] They are effective for mild to moderate pain associated with TMD. Aspirin (salicylate), which prevents prostaglandin synthesis, is the prototype for these compounds. All salicylate drugs are antipyretic, analgesic, and anti-inflammatory, but there are important differences in their effects. If the patient is sensitive to aspirin, a nonacetylated aspirin, choline magnesium trisalcylate (Trilisate) may be effective.[51] The therapeutic effect of opioid narcotics acts on specific opiate receptor sites in the central nervous system. These drugs have central nervous system depression qualities and addiction liabilities and depending on their potency may be used short-term for moderate to severe acute pain.

Nonsteroidal Anti-Inflammatory Drugs

Nonsteroidal anti-inflammatory drugs (NSAID) are effective against mild to moderate inflammatory conditions and postoperative pain. Their chief clinical application is as anti-inflammatory drugs in the treatment of musculoskeletal disorders. These drugs provide only symptomatic relief and do not arrest the progression of pathologic tissue injury except possibly in active inflammatory joint disease. Nonsteroidal anti-inflammatory drugs can be divided into two groups of compounds: (1) the indoles (of which indomethacin [Indocin] is the prototype), which include sulindac (Clinoril) and tolmetin sodium (Tolectin); and (2) propionic acid derivatives with a shorter half-life (eg, ibuprofen [Motrin], naproxen [Naprosyn], and fenoprofen [Nalfon]).

Corticosteroids

Although effective because of their anti-inflammatory effects, corticosteroids are not commonly prescribed for systemic use in the treatment of inflammation associated with TMD except for acute, generalized muscle and joint inflammation associated with polyarthritides. Intracapsular TMJ injection of corticosteroids (ie, methylprednisolone) has been recommended on a limited basis in cases of acute exacerbation of severe joint pain where conservative treatment has been unsuccessful.[52,53] It is thought that the drug effect causes more rapid resolution of symptoms, thus avoiding surgery in some cases. Conversely, it has been reported that injection of corticosteroids into the TMJ does not result in sustained improvement and that repeated injections are not effective in treating degenerative TMJ arthritis and may even accelerate joint degeneration.[45] Still others report significant short-term improvement with intracapsular injection of corticosteroids in patients with rheumatoid arthritis[54] and with no long-term sequelae.[55]

Muscle Relaxants

Muscle relaxants are prescribed to help prevent the increased muscle activity associated with TMD.[56] Mephenesin is the prototype for the majority of the oral skeletal muscle relaxants—the propanediols (eg, carisoprodol [Soma], methocarbamol [Robaxin], and chemically related chloroxazome [Paraflex, Parafon]). Experimentally, muscle relaxants depress spinal polysynaptic reflexes preferentially over monosynaptic reflexes. These compounds affect neuronal activity associated with muscle stretch reflexes, primarily in the lateral reticular area of the brainstem. The oral doses of all of these drugs are well below the amount required to elicit muscle relaxant activity experimentally; thus, some investigators conclude that their muscle relaxant activity is related only to their sedative effect.[57] Another commonly prescribed muscle relaxant, cyclobenzaprine (Flexeril), is similar to the structurally related tricyclic antidepressants in its effects. It is reported to act primarily at the brain stem level with the net effect of reduced tonic autonomic motor activity.[58] Some central skeletal muscle relaxants are available in combination with analgesics (eg, carisoprodol with phenacetin and caffeine [Soma Compound], chlorzoxazone with acetaminophen [Parafon Forte], methocarbamol with aspirin [Robaxisal]).

Antidepressants

The tertiary tricyclic antidepressants, particularly amitriptyline (Elavil), have analgesic properties independent of an antidepressant effect and are prescribed for chronic pain patients who have pain, depression, and sleep disturbance.[59–61] The therapeutic benefit of these drugs is related to their ability to increase the availability of the biogenic amine serotonin at the synaptic junctions in the central nervous system. The tricyclic antidepressants are beneficial in dosages as low as 10 mg in the treatment of muscle contraction headache and musculoskeletal pain.[62] They decrease the number of awakenings, increase stage IV (delta) sleep, and markedly decrease time in rapid eye movement (REM) sleep. For these reasons, they may have potential in the treatment of certain types of nocturnal bruxism. In dosages of 10 through 75 mg, the tricyclics are beneficial in the treatment of chronic orofacial pain and various oral dysaesthesias, which include glossodynia and idiopathic intraoral burning. When used as antidepressants, which requires an increase in therapeutic dosage, these drugs should only be prescribed by clinicians who have had special training in the diagnosis and treatment of depression.

Physical Therapy

Physical therapy helps to relieve musculoskeletal pain and to restore normal function by altering sensory input; reducing inflammation; decreasing, coordinating, and strengthening muscle activity; and promoting the repair and regeneration of tissues. In most cases, physical therapy is used as an adjunct to other treatments. Referral to and close cooperation with licensed professional therapists are recommended. Although well-controlled clinical trials have not been completed, physical therapy is well recognized as an effective, conservative method of treatment for TMD.[15,63–66]

Posture Training

The goal of posture training involves the prevention of untoward muscle activity of the head, neck, and shoulders, as well as the mandible and tongue. The aim should be to maintain orthostatic posture to prevent increased cervical and shoulder muscle activity and possible protrusion of the mandible. The posture of the tongue also effects the posture and function of the muscles attached to it. The more anterior the head is to the spinal column the greater is its effective weight. Except during function, the mandible should be in a relaxed (rest) position so that there is separation between the maxillary and mandibular teeth (prevents occlusal contact) and the tongue should rest gently on the anterior palate (prevents lateral tongue bracing). Although posture training is a common physical therapeutic approach, its relationship to TMD is not well understood and needs further study.

Exercise

Clinical experience suggests that an active exercise program is important to the development and maintenance of normal muscle and joint comfort, function, and stability. One of the objectives of an exercise program is to teach the patient how to avoid activities that are injurious to the synovial joints involved. In addition, exercise may be recommended to stretch and relax muscles,[67] increase joint range of motion, increase muscle strength, develop normal coordination arthrokinematics, and stabilize the TMJs. Three types of exercise are generally recommended: (1) repetitive exercises to establish coordinated, rhythmic muscle function; (2) isotonic exercises to increase range of motion; and (3) isometric exercises to increase muscular strength. They are prescribed to achieve specific goals and are changed or modified as the patient progresses. Most patients will not exercise if it increases pain; therefore, the therapist must initially help the patient to achieve some symptom relief with physical agents or modalities. A maintenance level of exercise is recommended to ensure long-term resolution once the patient has reached the goals of the treatment.

Mobilization

Mobilization techniques are indicated for decreased range of motion and pain due to muscle contracture, disc displacement without reduction, and fibrous adhesions in the joint. In some cases repeated manipulation by the therapist can restore a more physiologic length of resting muscle or improve joint function to permit a more normal range of motion.[68] Muscle relaxation and pain reduction are often required before mobilization can be effective. Thus, a combination of heat, cold, ultrasound, and electrical stimulation is often employed before or in conjunction with mobilization. Acute disc displacement without reduction at times can be effectively reduced by manipulation of the mandible, again usually after the use of physical agents and at times with the use of local anesthetic injections.[69] The mandible is gripped firmly with the clinician's thumbs on the occlusal surfaces of the posterior teeth, the unaffected side is securely braced, and the affected side is forced downward, forward, and inward.

Another technique incorporates the patient's voluntary maximal lateral excursive jaw movement to the nonaffected side followed by opening through the lateral border movement.[70] Arthrographic studies indicate that manipulation does not produce complete anatomic reduction of the disc but does increase disc mobilization.[71] Following mobilization, therapy to maintain the reduced condyle-disc relation should be considered, such as orthopedic appliance therapy, relaxation therapy, and exercises.

The application of continuous passive motion for postsurgical therapy has recently been implemented by oral and maxillofacial surgeons.[72,73] It is reasonable to suggest that there are the same indications and advantages for its use following TMJ surgery as with orthopedic surgery in general.

Physical Agents or Modalities

Physical agents or modalities for TMD management include electrotherapy and ultrasound modalities, anesthetic agents, and acupuncture. Electrotherapy devices that produce thermal, histochemical, and physiologic changes in the muscles and joint are divided into high-voltage stimulation (electrogalvanic stimulation [EGS]), low-voltage stimulation (transcutaneous electrical nerve stimulation [TENS]), and microvoltage stimulation. Electrogalvanic stimulation uses a high-voltage, low-amperage, monophasic current of varying frequencies. This modality produces a reduction of muscle pain and activity and enhances healing.[74] Transcutaneous electrical nerve stimulation uses a low-voltage, low-amperage, biphasic current at varying frequencies and is designed primarily for sensory counter stimulation in painful disorders.[75] Like EGS, this modality decreases muscle pain and hyperactivity and also can be an aid in muscle re-education. If significant motor stimulation occurs concurrently, this may impair the analgesic effect and even exacerbate acute pain.[76] Microcurrent electrical stimulation is reputed to apply a microvoltage at the approximate electrochemical spectrum that occurs neurophysiologically at the synaptic junction. It has been used primarily for pain relief. To date, only clinical evidence has suggested the use of electrical stimulation for the treatment of pain related to TMD.

Ultrasound is a frequently used physical treatment modality in physical medicine for musculoskeletal problems. With ultrasound, the high-frequency oscillations of the transducer head are converted to heat when transmitted through the tissue. This can heat to a depth of 5 cm and may decrease the convalescence period associated with painful joint disorders. Ultrasound is used to produce deep heat in the joints, to treat joint contracture by increasing the stretch of the extracapsular soft tissue, to decrease chronic pain, muscle contraction, and tendonitis, and to facilitate resorption of calcium deposits with bursitis.[77–82] The potentially critical parameters of ultrasound such as duration of treatment, number of sessions, exposure time per session, frequency, and intensity need further systematic study.[83]

Anesthetic agents can also be beneficial to TMD therapy. Application of vapocoolant sprays followed by muscle stretching decreases muscle soreness and tightness and is thought to inactivate myofascial trigger points.[84,85] The spray is applied to the affected area from approximately an 18-inch working distance in a sweeping motion in the direction of the muscle fibers. The eyes, ears, and nasal mucosa must be protected. Local anesthetic injections, alone or in conjunction with muscle stretching or mobilization, also have been shown to be useful for myofascial trigger point management.[86]

Once muscle pain cycles are interrupted with local anesthetic injections, relief may last beyond the duration of the anesthetic. Procaine (1.0% to 2.0% without epinephrine diluted to 0.5% with sterile saline) is recommended for trigger point injections because it is thought to be the least myotoxic local anesthetic.[87]

Acupuncture has also been used for the treatment of chronic pain. The therapeutic effects of acupuncture on pain and dysfunction are usually explained by neural and humoral pathways.[88] In a randomized study comparing acupuncture and conventional treatment modalities in the management of TMD,[89] the patients surveyed favored conventional therapy; however, there was no statistical difference in pain relief or improvement in function. Another random, controlled study had the same positive results as acupuncture.[90] Further study of this approach for TMD is indicated.

Orthopedic Appliance Therapy

Orthopedic appliances, commonly referred to as interocclusal splints, orthotics, nightguards, or bruxism appliances, are routinely used in the treatment of TMD. Removable acrylic resin appliances that cover the teeth have been used to alter occlusal relationships and to redistribute occlusal forces,[91,92] to prevent wear and mobility of the teeth,[93,94] to reduce bruxism and parafunction,[22,95] to treat masticatory muscle pain and dysfunction,[26,96–99] and to alter structural relationships in the TMJ.[68,100–103]

The reduction of painful symptoms with appliance therapy has been well documented. Many studies have found resolution of symptoms after insertion of an appliance.[26,99,104–107] Clark[26] reviewed the design, theory, and effectiveness of orthopedic appliances for specific symptoms and found a 70% to 90% rate of clinical success. Although the treatment effect was predictable, the physiologic basis of the treatment response has not been well understood.

The complications that can occur with the excessive or incorrect use of any appliance include caries, gingival inflammation, mouth odors, speech difficulties, tooth-contact relation changes, and psychologic dependence on the appliance. Serious complications include major irreversible changes in the interocclusal or interarch relation as a result of long-term use of all appliances, and particularly with the partial-arch coverage appliances.[108] Appliances must not be designed to allow or provide for tooth movement during active treatment of TMD signs and symptoms. There are many useful types of appliances; but two major types of appliances, stabilization appliances and anterior positioning appliances, are commonly used for TMD management.

Stabilization Appliances

Stabilization appliances, also termed "flat plane", "gnathologic", or "muscle relaxation splints", should cover all of the mandibular or maxillary teeth. They are designed to provide joint stabilization, protect the teeth, redistribute forces, relax the elevator muscles, and decrease bruxism.[22,26,91,97,106,107,109–115] Wearing the appliance increases the patient's awareness of jaw habits and helps alter the posture of the mandible to a more open, relaxed (rest) position. Electromyographic monitoring of the masseter muscle has shown a short-term decrease in the level of bruxism activity when an appliance is worn.[22,116,117] In another study, appliance therapy decreased muscle activity in approximately 50% of the treated patients; however, it increased muscle activity in approximately 30% of the patients.[96] Recent EMG studies have documented a short-term reduction in elevator muscle activity and a short-term increase in suprahyoid muscle activity.[118,119]

The occlusal surface of the appliance should be adjusted to provide a stable physiologic mandibular posture by creating bilateral, even posterior occlusal contacts for the opposing teeth on closure. Anterior guidance is usually provided by acrylic guide ramps in the canine or anterior areas of the appliance to separate the opposing posterior teeth from the appliance in all lateral, lateroprotrusive, and protrusive excursions of the mandible. Clinical experience suggests that the occlusal surface of the appliance should be adjusted initially and periodically to compensate for changes in the maxillomandibular relation as pain, muscle activity, inflammation, edema, or soft tissue structural relations change.

The protocol should be monitored on a timely basis for the initial period until the maxillomandibular relation stabilizes.[120] In acute cases, the appliance is usually best worn full time for a specified period of time. As resolution occurs, use of the appliance only at night can be considered. Recently a study suggested that nocturnal appliance use only was more successful in patients with muscle disorders, whereas patients with articular disorders benefited from continuous appliance use (24-hour wear).[121] Eventually, intermittent use at night during periods of increased stressful life events should suffice, if the appliance is needed at all. Ideally, the patient should eliminate full-time use of an appliance. Patients not showing a positive response within 3 to 4 weeks should be reevaluated. Failure to show an initial positive response does not mandate more aggressive or prolonged therapy; rather, other factors should be considered: chronic pain behavior, noncompliance, misdiagnosis, or degree of tissue pathology.

If a stabilizing appliance is fabricated with a soft resilient material, it should be used on a temporary basis when worn full time or it should only be worn part time. Full-time wear can result in uncontrolled changes in tooth position due to the dimensional instability of the soft appliance. The efficacy of resilient appliances for decreasing bruxism and TMD signs and symptoms is not clear.[116,122,123]

Anterior Positioning Appliances

Anterior positioning appliances, also termed mandibular orthopedic repositioning appliances (MORAs), are used to decrease joint pain, joint noise (clicking), and associated secondary muscle symptoms in TMD.[101,102,124–128] Anterior positioning appliances may effect the TMJ in two ways: (1) they may decrease adverse loading (compression) in the joint, and (2) they may alter the structural condyle-disc relation. The primary indication for anterior positioning appliance therapy is acute joint pain associated with joint noise, intermittent locking, and/or structural bony changes.[102,125,129–134] Prior to this approach, the occlusal consequences should be determined and discussed with the patient because mandibular repositioning can result in irreversible changes in the occlusion (ie, posterior open bite). For a number of patients a stabilization appliance can accomplish many of the same goals as can an anterior positioning appliance with less risk of irreversible consequences and, thus, should be considered first.

Anterior positioning appliances are fabricated for either dental arch to cover the occlusal surfaces of all teeth with occlusal indentations, guide ramps, or both that cause the mandible to temporarily advance or protrude into a therapeutic (ie, less painful) condyle-disc-fossa relation. An anterior positioning appliance is most efficient for decompression of the joint when it is worn full time at the beginning of treatment. However, part-time use at night is effective for preventing intermittent disc displacement without reduction on awakening, with less potential for the occlusal consequences of full-time use. The appliance should initially be adjusted for occlusal stability in as minimal an anterior mandibular position as possible (2 mm or less) to decrease the pain and dysfunction. Once joint pain and dysfunction (ie, intermittent locking) are decreased, the appliance should be adjusted to, or replaced with, a stabilization appliance to allow posterior repositioning of the mandible to the approximate pretreatment occlusal position. The appliance should be adjusted back to this more physiologic stable position within a 6- to 12-week period. This approach is strongly recommended to avoid or minimize the need for unnecessary restorative, prosthodontic, or orthodontic therapy.

Although short-term success with anterior positioning appliances is good,[103,126,134] long-term use is not encouraging.[129,134] Because constant long-term use of an anterior positioning appliance can create iatrogenic occlusal problems, anterior positioning should be attempted only in selected cases of articular pain and if the patient understands the possible treatment consequences. If anterior positioning is not a viable option, a stabilization splint with adjunctive therapy for pain relief and improved function is indicated.[135] Although clicking is not usually eliminated, it may be decreased, and asymptomatic clicks, by themselves, do not warrant treatment. If the anterior positioning appliance approach does not affect satisfactorily the patient's internal derangement and significant pain or limited range of motion continues, arthroscopy or surgical repair of the disc may be necessary or definitive changes in the occlusion with dental treatment may be required.

Occlusal Therapy

The topic of occlusion continues to remain an enigma to those interested in studying therapeutic concepts and TMD pathophysiology related to occlusal discrepancies. It is difficult to establish any significant cause and effect relationships due to the many variables involved, some of which are difficult, if not impossible, to exclude clinically.[48,136] To be sure, there are many valid reasons for treatment of the occlusion for numerous dental conditions (ie, lack of interarch/intra-arch tooth stability; tooth mobility; fremitus; occlusion-related tooth or restoration fracture; tooth sensitivity; altered or compromised masticatory function, swallowing, or speech; and compromised supporting tissues due to adverse loading). Although dental treatment may be necessary for patients with TMD, it is believed to be infrequently necessary for the purpose of direct treatment for TMD.

Primary occlusal therapy should be used with caution because there is little evidence that natural occlusal morphologic variation is a cause of TMD.[137,138] Because most occlusal features previously associated with TMD now appear to have minimal scientific relationship to clinical signs and symptoms, the appropriateness of treatment emphasis on the correction of chronic malocclusion is becoming questionable.[137,138] Yet, in spite of the fact that a strong correlation between occlusal morphology and TMD treatment outcome has not been shown,[139] dentists continue to consider occlusal therapy necessary for definitive treatment of TMD.[140] Recently it has been cited that treatment directed to the correction of a chronic or adapted malocclusion or occlusal variation may be appropriate because it can be a symptom rather than a cause of TMD.[137,138] A wide variety of segments of the stomatognathic system may occur

as biologically successful adaptation and are not necessarily pathognomic.[141] Thus, any occlusomorphologic explanations for TMD should be resisted until the TMD have stabilized and there is reasonable assurance that further occlusal changes will not occur.[120,142]

When considering occlusal changes in the TMD patient, the clinician is advised to proceed cautiously, using the least invasive procedures possible, with constant patient reassessment.[143] Occlusal alteration in TMD patients should be minimized (ie, the pretreatment intercuspal relationship and condylar position should be preserved whenever possible) after they have received treatment for TMD. There is no evidence that anterior guidance is superior to other forms of guidance for treating TMD symptoms related to nocturnal bruxism, as studied with orthopedic appliances,[144,145] or that it would provide the optimum joint loading for all TMD articular conditions.[146,147] In general, there is a lack of evidence that the composition of an idealized occlusion through complex occlusal therapy is necessary for TMD management.[138,148]

Occlusal Adjustment

Occlusal adjustment for TMD has been recommended as beneficial,[149] but more recently this treatment has been shown not to be as effective as the more conservative modalities in reducing TMD symptoms and headache.[150] For that reason, occlusal adjustment as an irreversible treatment modality should rarely be considered as a primary component of TMD treatment. Limited occlusal adjustment may be appropriate in primary treatment stages when intercuspal position (ICP) relationships provoke acute symptomatology,[151] ie, when acute symptoms result from interferences following recent restorative dental treatments. Occlusal adjustment may also be considered for enhanced mandibular stability and for redistribution of adverse loading forces in cases where a specific TMD disturbance has resulted in an unstable occlusal relation. For example, a skeletal anterior open bite development may occur following an aggressive TMJ arthritic condition.[137,152] With regard to bruxism, there is no evidence that prophylactic selective grinding of occlusal surfaces is beneficial or that it eliminates bruxism.[1,105] Occlusal adjustment is never indicated for prevention of TMD.[153] There may be an indication for occlusal adjustment, however, in conjunction with a coexisting dental treatment need, such as stabilization of postorthodontic-postorthognathic therapy or finalization of reconstructive dental therapy.[154]

Restorative Therapy

Some questions have been posed regarding the benefits of occlusal restorative care for TMD patients.[155] As with other kinds of irreversible treatment, restorative therapy should never be primary but may follow initial resolution of TMD symptoms and dysfunctional instability. However, once stability and symptom resolution are achieved, restorative therapy can be considered in those patients who are likely to benefit from reduction of adverse loading and improvement of occlusal force redistribution, as suggested by studies of Hannam,[156] Hylander,[157] and Faulkner et al.[158] However, the scientific basis for the belief that occlusal factors influence loading within the TMJ or cause TMD is weak at best. With this in mind there are, however, instances when the dental consequences of TMD results in functional mandibular instability that must be addressed.

Extensive restorative therapy should be undertaken with caution because the speed of change with treatment carries some risk in TMD patients[142]; however, the risk in TMD patients as a group appears to be minimal.[159] Altered occlusal relations can advantageously redistribute loading forces but disturb existing stable conditions elsewhere in the masticatory system.[111] It is possible, therefore, that symptoms may be exacerbated if the demand for adaptation is beyond the adaptive capacity of the tissues or if the TMD patient is already functioning at the limit of his or her adaptive range.

Orthodontic-Orthognathic Therapy

When major occlusal alterations are considered to be advantageous dentally, orthodontic therapy is often the treatment of choice because it is less invasive than is extensive reconstructive therapy. Fixed, removable, functional, and extraoral appliances are all capable of improving occlusal and mandibular stability.[160,161] Frequently, orthodontic therapy is recommended to provide occlusal support following anterior repositioning therapy. However, this has not proven to be as successful on a longitudinal basis when compared to anterior positioning splint therapy alone.[129,162] Orthodontic therapy, even with the normally healthy patient, but in particular with the TMD patient, presents some risk of destabilizing the stomatognathic system during treatment.[163] Hence, the orthodontic diagnosis and treatment plan must reflect possible influences of occlusal instabilities created during treatment with pre-existing joint pathology, trauma associated disease, and anatomic variations.[26,164–166]

However, recent retrospective clinical studies have reported no greater prevalence of TMD signs or symptoms in highly selective samples of postorthodontic subjects than in untreated subjects of similar ages.[167-181] Furthermore, other studies comparing postorthodontic patients with and without premolar extractions found no differences in posttreatment condylar position,[182-185] overbite,[184] discrepancy between intercuspal position and retruded contact position,[186] mandibular position,[187] or in overall TMD symptomatology.[181,188,189]

A recent study concluded that it cannot be ruled out that some patients acquire a more posterior location of the condyle during correction of any Class II, Division I malocclusion with extraction only of maxillary premolars, but the prevalence was similar to controls shortly after therapy.[190] A few studies have found a higher incidence of joint sounds (clicking) on a longitudinal basis, especially with premolar extraction; however, it was possibly explained by the original growth pattern more than by the extractions because the clicking predated the actual treatment.[176,191] There are some longitudinal studies that, in fact, show that subjects with a history of orthodontic treatment tend to have a lower prevalence of TMD signs and symptoms than do control groups who have not had orthodontic therapy.[170,188,192]

Although as a group there is little evidence that orthodontically treated patients have greater prevalence of TMD symptoms, the individual response to the dental instabilities associated with orthodontic treatment may be quite different. Thus, the practitioner must be alert for, and be prepared to deal with, the onset or exacerbation of signs and symptoms for whatever reason they may occur during orthodontic tooth movement.[160] This potential clearly mandates a pretreatment screening examination of all orthodontic patients for asymptomatic signs.[193]

Orthognathic surgery may be considered in conjunction with orthodontic or restorative treatment for correction of major structural mandibular deformities, discrepancies, or instabilities. However, orthognathic surgery should only be contemplated in TMD patients following careful evaluation after all symptoms have been reasonably resolved and the maxillomandibular relation has been stabilized. Surgical treatment for skeletal asymmetries and growth anomalies with the specific intent of alleviating *pain* associated with TMD is very questionable at this time. But in those TMD patients with severe skeletal malocclusion who may benefit from greater dental-skeletal stability, orthognathic surgery in conjunction with orthodontic therapy is often the method of choice.[175,194-196]

Surgery

Temporomandibular surgery has become an effective treatment for specific articular disorders. However, the complexity of available techniques, potential for complications, frequency of behavioral and psychosocial contributing factors, and the availability of nonsurgical approaches, make TMJ surgery an approach that should be used only in selected cases.

The decision to treat the patient surgically depends on the degree of pathology or anatomic derangement present within the joint, the repairability of that condition, the results of appropriate nonsurgical therapy, and the extent of impairment that the joint pathology creates for the patient. The appropriate duration and complexity of nonsurgical therapy before considering surgery are determined by a combination of factors including the expected prognosis compared with the actual patient improvement, the degree of impairment, and the patient's compliance with the program. Patients with complicating factors such as litigation, depression, or uncontrolled nocturnal bruxism may have a poor surgical prognosis. In addition, the clinician must have a full knowledge and appreciation of the potential complications and the potential for surgical failure. Once this information is available, a realistic discussion of the prognosis, the patient's expectations, and the complicating factors can help a patient to make the correct decision about surgery.

Preoperative and postoperative nonsurgical management must be integrated into the overall surgical treatment plan.[197] This therapy is directed toward decreasing the functional load placed on the joint, eliminating or modifying contributing factors such as oral parafunctional habits, and providing appropriate psychologic and medical support. The following criteria adapted from The American Association of Oral and Maxillofacial Surgeons[198] should be addressed before proceeding with TMJ surgery: (1) documented TMJ internal derangement or other structural joint disorder with appropriate imaging; (2) positive evidence to suggest that the symptoms and objective findings are a result of a structural disorder; (3) pain and/or dysfunction of such magnitude as to constitute a disability to the patient; (4) prior unsuccessful nonsurgical treatment; (5) prior management, to the extent possible, of bruxism, oral parafunctional habits, other medical or dental conditions, and other contributing factors that may affect the outcome of surgery; and (6) patient consent after a discussion of potential complications, goals to achieve, success rate, timing, postoperative management, and alternative approaches including no treatment. These conditions maximize the potential for a successful outcome but cannot guarantee it. Surgical management may include closed surgical procedures (arthroscopy) and open surgical procedures (arthrotomy).

Arthroscopy

Arthroscopy holds promise for histopathologic and biochemical sampling of the joint tissues[199] and as a modality for treating painful joint hypomobility secondary to a persistent nonreducing displaced disc or arthrosis.[200–203] Arthroscopic revision of previous open surgery has also been helpful in alleviating postoperative pain and intracapsular fibrosis.[204] At this time, the arthroscope is used mainly to examine the upper joint space, and surgery is limited to biopsies, minor debridement and lavage, and incising minor adhesions within the upper joint space.[205] Recent evidence reveals that reduction of symptoms following arthroscopic surgery is not due to improved disc position or joint sounds and that any inferred long-term benefits are still undetermined at this time.[206,207] Postoperative MRI scans reveal that following arthroscopic procedures a vast majority of patients have persistent anterior displacement but increased disc mobility.[208–212] Further, it has been suggested that simple irrigation or lavage (arthrocentesis) with or without intra-articular corticosteroids and manipulation may be as effective as arthroscopic lavage.[213]

Arthrotomy

Open surgical intervention of the TMJ (arthrotomy) usually is required for bony or fibrous ankylosis, neoplasia, severe chronic dislocations, persistent painful disc derangement, and severe osteoarthrosis refractory to conservative modalities of treatment. Surgery is less often indicated in displaced condylar fractures, agenesis of the condyle, and severe, painful, chronic arthritides. Surgery is seldom, if ever, indicated in inflammatory joint disorders (synovitis or capsulitis), condylysis, and nonpainful degenerative arthritis. Thus, arthrotomy is generally indicated for the patient with advanced disease who meets the surgical criteria or who has disease refractory to or not amenable to arthroscopic surgical techniques.

Open joint surgical procedures may range from discoplasty, discal repositioning, or discectomy with or without replacement to arthroplasty, which includes high condylectomy. Discoplasty and disc repositioning with plication has been reported to have an 80% to 90% success rate.[214] Discectomy (meniscectomy) is performed with[215,216] or without autogenous or homologous replacement.[217] However, the recent trend is either not to replace the disc at all or to use a vascularized flap (ie, temporalis muscle and fascia) to maintain structural relationships.[218,219] Due to the long-term complications with alloplastic prostheses for disc replacement, their use is contraindicated and even temporary use is questioned.[220–226] In fact, the December 1991 issue of the Food and Drug Administration Medical Bulletin[227] regarding serious problems with proplast-coated TMJ implants (implant perforation, fragmentation and/or foreign body response resulting in progressive bone degeneration) has recommended immediate and appropriate clinical and radiographic examination of all previous implant patients, with re-examination once a year to include CT or MRI scans. Removal of the implant is recommended if "progressive bone degeneration or implant disruption is found or if pain or occlusal changes persist 6 months or longer."

Arthroplasty is indicated for recontouring of the articular surfaces with or without removal of the disc. High condylectomy minimizes postsurgical sequelae and, when the disc is maintained, eliminates mechanical interference to the disc.[228] Condylectomy and subcondylar osteotomy (condylotomy) are performed infrequently; they are indicated for more complex disease or traumatic conditions.[229,230]

There can be more postsurgical sequelae, including marked occlusal changes, with these procedures. The outcome criteria of assessing surgery results are based on the patient's report of decreased intensity or infrequency of pain, increased jaw function and range of motion (vertical incisal opening to at least 35 mm), and the ability for the patient to return to a normal lifestyle, which includes a normal diet.

References

1. Greene CS, Laskin DM: Long term evaluation of treatment for myofascial pain-dysfunction syndrome: A comparative analysis. J Am Dent Assoc 1983;107:235–238.

2. Mejersjö C, Carlsson GE: Long term results of treatment for temporomandibular pain-dysfunction. J Prosthet Dent 1983;49:809–815.

3. Fricton JR: Recent advances in temporomandibular disorders and orofacial pain. J Am Dent Assoc 1991;122:25–32.

4. Fricton JR: Clinical care for myofascial pain. Dent Clin North Am 1991;35:1–28.

5. Carlsson GE: Long-term effects of treatment of craniomandibular disorders. J Craniomand Pract 1985;3:337–342.

6. Randolph CS, Greene CS, Moretti R, Forbes D, Perry HT: Conservative management of temporomandibular disorders: A posttreatment comparison between patients from a university clinic and from private practice. Am J Orthod Dentofac Orthop 1990;98:77–82.

7. Apfelberg DB, Lovey E, Janetos G, Maser MR, Lash H: Temporomandibular joint disease. Results of a ten-year study. Post-Grad Med 1979;65:167–172.

8. Okeson JP, Hayes DK: Long-term results of treatment for temporomandibular disorders: An evaluation by patients. J Am Dent Assoc 1986;112:473–478.

9. Helkimo E, Westling L: History, clinical

findings, and outcome of treatment of patients with anterior disk displacement. J Craniomand Pract 1987;5:270–276.

10. Rasmussen OC: Description of population and progress of symptoms in a longitudinal study of temporomandibular arthropathy. Scand J Dent Res 1981;89: 196–203.

11. Nickerson JW, Boering G: Natural course of osteoarthrosis as it related to internal derangement of the temporomandibular joint. Oral Maxillofac Surg Clin North Am 1989;1:27–45.

12. Flor H, Fydrich T, Turk DC: Efficacy of multidisciplinary pain treatment centers: a meta-analytic review. Pain 1992;49:221–230.

13. Hodges JM: Managing temporomandibular joint syndrome. Laryngoscope 1990; 100:60–66.

14. Howard JA, Lovrovich AT: Wind instruments: Their interplay with orofacial structures. Med Probl Perform Arts 1989; 4:59–72.

15. Danzig W, VanDyke AR: Physical therapy as an adjunct to temporomandibular joint therapy. J Prosthet Dent 1983;49: 96–99.

16. Rugh JD: Behavioral therapy. In Mohl ND, Zarb GA, Carlsson GE and Rugh JD (eds) A Textbook in Occlusion. Chicago, Quintessence Publ Co, 1988, pp 329–338.

17. Melamed RG, Mealiea WL Jr: Behavioral intervention in pain-related problems in dentistry. In Ferguson JM, Taylor CB (eds) The Comprehensive Handbook of Behavioral Medicine. Vol 2. New York, Spectrum Inc, 1981, pp 241–259.

18. Mealiea WL, McGlynn D: Temporomandibular disorders and bruxism. In Hatch JP, Fisher JG, Rugh JD (eds) Biofeedback Studies in Clinical Efficacy. New York, Plenum Press, 1987 pp 123–151.

19. Rugh JD: Psychological components of pain. Dent Clin North Am 1987;31:579–594.

20. Cannistraci AJ, Fritz G: Dental applications of biofeedback. In JV Basmajiam (ed) Biofeedback, Principles and Practice for Clinicians. Baltimore, Williams and Wilkins, 1989, pp 297–310.

21. Solberg WK, Rugh JD: The use of biofeedback devices in the treatment of bruxism. South Calif Dent Assoc J 1972;40: 852–853.

22. Solberg WK, Clark GT, Rugh JD: Nocturnal electromyographic evaluation of bruxism patients undergoing short term splint therapy. J Oral Rehabil 1975;2: 215–223.

23. Kardachi BJ, Bailey JO, Ash MM: A comparison of biofeedback and occlusal adjustment on bruxism. J Periodontol 1978; 48:639–642.

24. Rugh JD, Johnson RW: Temporal analysis of nocturnal bruxism during EMG feedback. J Periodontol 1981;52:263–265.

25. Pierce CJ, Gale EN: A comparison of different treatments for nocturnal bruxism. J Dent Res 1988;67:597–601.

26. Clark GT: A critical evaluation of orthopedic interocclusal appliance therapy: Design, theory, and overall effectiveness. J Am Dent Assoc 1984;108:359–364.

27. Levinson NA: Psychologic facets of esthetic dental health care: A developmental perspective. J Prosthet Dent 1990;64: 486–491.

28. Sandler J, Dare C: The psychoanalytic concept of orality. J Psychosom Res 1970; 14:211–222.

29. Barsky AJ, Klerman GL: Overview: Hypochondriasis, bodily complaints and somatic styles. Am J Psychiatry 1983;140: 273–283.

30. Lipowski ZJ: Somatization: The concept and its clinical application. Am J Psychiatry 1988;145:1358–1368.

31. Brown HN, Vaillant GE: Hypochondriasis. Arch Int Med 1981;141:723–726.

32. Nemiah JC, Sifneos PC: Affect and fantasy in patients with psychosomatic disorders. In Hill O (ed) Modern Trends in Psychosomatic Medicine, Vol 2, London, Butterworth Publ, 1970, pp 26–34.

33. Wahl CW: Unconscious factors in the psychodynamics of the hypochondriacal patient. Psychosomatics 1963;4:9–14.

34. Katon W: Panic disorder and somatization. Am J Med 1984;77:101–106.

35. Nemiah JC: Alexithymia. Psychother Psychosom 1977;28:199–206.

36. Turk DC, Salovey P: Chronic pain as a variant of depressive disease: A critical reappraisal. J Nerv Ment Dis 1984;172:398–404.

37. Quill TE: Somatization disorder. JAMA 1985;254:3075–3079.

38. Lipp M: Respectful Treatment. New York, Harper & Row Publ, Inc, 1977.

39. Quill TE: Partnerships in patient care: A contractual approach. Ann Intern Med 1983;98:228–234.

40. Sternbach RA: Pain Patients: Traits and Treatment. New York, Academic Press, 1974.

41. Fordyce WE: On opioids and treatment targets. Am Pain Soc Bull 1991;1:1–34.

42. Jaffe JH, Martin JR: Analgesics and antagonists. In Goodman and Gilman (eds) The Pharmacologic Basis of Therapeutics. 7th ed. New York, McMillan, 1985, pp 491–532.

43. Ready LB, Hare B: Drug problems in chronic pain patients. Anesthesiol Rev 1979;6:28–31.

44. Turk DC, Brody MC: Chronic opioid therapy for persistent noncancer pain: Panacea or oxymoron? Am Pain Soc Bull 1992;1:4–7.

45. Gangarosa LP, Mahan PE: Pharmacologic management of TMJ-MPDS. Ear Nose Throat J 1982;61:30–41.

46. Gregg JM: Pharmacological management of myofascial pain dysfunction. In Laskin D, Greenfield W, Gale E, Rugh J, Neff P, et al (eds) The President's Conference on the Examination, Diagnosis, and Management of Temporomandibular Disorders. Chicago, American Dental Association, 1983; pp 167–173.

47. Gregg JM, Rugh JD: Pharmacological therapy. In Mohl ND, Zarb GA, Carlsson GE, Rugh JD (eds) A Textbook on Occlusion. Chicago, Quintessence Publ Co, 1988, pp 351–375.

48. McNeill C: Temporomandibular disorders: Guidelines for diagnosis and management. J Calif Dent Assoc 1991;19:15–26.

49. Levine JD, Gordon NC, Smith R, McBryde B: Desipramine enhances opiate postoperative analgesic. Pain 1986; 27:45–49.

50. Flower JR, Moncada S, Vane JR: Drug therapy of inflammation. In Goodman and Gilman (eds) The Pharmacologic Basis of Therapeutics. 7th ed. New York, McMillan, 1985, pp 674–716.

51. Tanaka TT: Differential diagnosis of arthritic disorders: Appendix, Management of arthritic disorders with pharmaceuticals. Topics Geriatric Rehab 1990;5:47–49.

52. Toller P: Osteoarthritis of the mandibular condyle. Br Dent J 1973;134:223–231.

53. Wenneberg B, Kopp S: Short term effect of intra-articular injections of corticosteroid on temporomandibular pain and dysfunction. Swed Dent J 1978;2:189–196.

54. Kopp S, Åkerman S, Nilner M: Short-term effects of intra-articular sodium hyaluronate, glucocorticoid, and saline injections on rheumatoid arthritis of the temporomandibular joint. J Craniomandib Disord Facial Oral Pain 1991;5:231–238.

55. Wenneberg B, Kopp S, Grondahl H-G: Long term effect of intra-articular injections of a glucocorticosteroid into the TMJ: A clinical and radiographic 8-year follow-up. J Craniomandib Disord Facial Oral Pain 1991;5:11–18.

56. Stanko JR: A review of oral skeletal muscle relaxants for the craniomandibular disorder (CMD) practitioner. J Craniomand Pract 8:234–243.

57. Smith CM: Skeletal muscle relaxants. In Smith CM, Reynard AM (eds) Textbook of Pharmacology. Philadelphia, WB Saunders Co, 1992, pp 358–366.

58. Gatter RA: Pharmacotherapeutics in fibrositis. Am J Med 1986;81(suppl 3A):63–66.

59. Sharar Y, Singer E, Schmidt E, Dionne RA, Dubner R: The analgesic effect of amitriptyline on chronic facial pain. Pain 1987;31:199–209.

60. Brown RS, Bottomley WK: The utilization and mechanism of action of tricyclic antidepressants in the treatment of chronic facial pain: A review of the literature. Anesth Prog 1990;37:223–229.

61. Tura B, Tura SM: The analgesic effect of tricyclic antidepressants. Brain Res 1990;518:19–22.

62. Kreisberg MK: Tricyclic antidepressants: Analgesic effect and indications in orofacial pain. J Craniomandib Disord Facial Oral Pain 1988;2:171–177.

63. Friedman MH, Weisberg J: Temporomandibular Joint Disorders Diagnosis and Treatment. Chicago, Quintessence Publ Co, 1985, pp 124–140.

64. Solberg WK: Temporomandibular disorders: Masticatory myalgia and its management. Br Dent J 1986;160:351–356.

65. Kirk WS, Calabrese DK: Clinical evaluation of physical therapy in the management of internal derangement of the temporomandibular joint. J Oral Maxillofac Surg 1989;47:113–119.

66. Clark GT, Adachi NY, Dornan MR: Physical medicine procedures affect temporomandibular disorders: A review. J Am Dent Assoc 1990;121:151–161.

67. Carlson CR, Okeson JP, Falace DA, Nitz AJ, Anderson D: Stretch-based relaxation and the reduction of EMG activity among masticatory muscle pain patients. J Craniomandib Disord Facial Oral Pain 1991;5:205–212.

68. Farrar WB, McCarty WL Jr: A Clinical Outline of Temporomandibular Joint Diagnosis and Treatment. 7th ed. Montgomery, Normandie Publ, 1982, p 129.

69. Van Dyke A, Goldman SM: Manual reduction of displaced disc. Cranio 1990;8:350–352.

70. Minagi S, Nozaki S, Sato T, Tsuru H: A manipulation technique for treatment of anterior disk displacement without reduction. J Prosthet Dent 1991;65:686–691.

71. Segami N, Murakami K-I, Iizuka T, Fukuda M: Arthrographic evaluation of disk position following mandibular manipulation technique for internal derangement with closed-lock of the temporomandibular joint. J Craniomandib Disord Facial Oral Pain 1990;4:99–108.

72. Poremba EP, Moffett BC: The effect of continuous passive motion on the temporomandibular joint after surgery. Part I: Appliance design and fabrication. Oral Surg Oral Med Oral Pathol 1989;67:490–498.

73. Sebastian MH, Moffett BC: The effect on continuous passive motion on the temporomandibular joint after surgery. Part II: Appliance improvement, normal subject evaluation, pilot clinical trial. Oral Surg Oral Med Oral Pathol 1989;67:644–653.

74. Binder SA: Applications of low and high-voltage electrotherapeutic currents. In Wolf WL (ed) Electrotherapy. New York, Churchill Livingstone, 1981, pp 1–25.

75. Møystad A, Krogstad BS, Larheim TA: Transcutaneous nerve stimulation in a group of patients with rheumatic disease involving the temporomandibular joint. J Prosthet Dent 1990;64:596–600.

76. Mohl ND, Ohrbach RK, Crowe HC, Gross AJ: Devices for the diagnosis and treatment of temporomandibular disorders. Part III. Thermography ultrasound, electrical stimulation, and EMG biofeedback. J Prosthet Dent 1990;63:472–477.

77. Mannheimer JS: Therapeutic modalities. In Kraus, SL (ed) TMJ Disorders: Management of the Craniomandibular Complex. New York, Churchill Livingstone, 1988, pp 311–337.

78. McDiarmid T, Burns PN: Clinical applications of therapeutic ultrasound. Physiotherapy 1987;73:155–162.

79. Patrick MK: Applications of therapeutic pulsed ultrasound. Physiotherapy 1978;64:103–104.

80. Ruskin AF: Current Therapy in Physiatry. Philadelphia, WB Saunders Co, 1984.

81. Williams AR: Ultrasound: Biological Effects and Potential Hazards. New York, Academic Press, 1983.

82. Ziskin MC, Michlovitz SL: Therapeutic ultrasound. In Michlovitz SL (ed) Thermal Agents in Rehabilitation. Philadelphia, F A Davis Co, 1986, pp 141–176.

83. Hashish I, Harvey W, Harris M: Anti-inflammatory effects of ultrasound therapy: Evidence for a major placebo effect. Br J Rheumatol 1986;25:77–81.

84. Travell JG, Simons DG: Myofascial Pain and Dysfunction: The Trigger Point Manual. Baltimore, Williams and Wilkins, 1983, pp 63–74.

85. Jaeger B, Reeves JL: Quantification of changes in myofascial trigger point sensitivity with pressure algometer following passive stretch. Pain 1986;27:203–210.

86. Jaeger B, Skootsky SA: Double blind controlled study of different myofascial trigger point injection techniques. Pain 1987; 4(suppl):abstr 560.

87. Ritchie JM, Greene NM: Local anesthetics. In Goodman and Gilman (eds) The Pharmacologic Basis of Therapeutics. 7th ed. New York, McMillan, 1985, pp 302–322.

88. Bannerman RH: The World Health Organization viewpoint on acupuncture. World Health Organization, Geneva, 1979.

89. Raustia AM, Pohjola RT, Virtanen KK: Acupuncture compared with stomatognathic treatment for TMJ dysfunction. Part I. A randomized study. J Prosthet Dent 1985;54:581–585.

90. Johansson A, Wenneberg B, Wagersten C, Haraldson T: Acupuncture in treatment of facial muscular pain. Acta Odontol Scand 1991;49:153–158.

91. Ramfjord SP, Ash MM: Occlusion. 3rd ed. Philadelphia, WB Saunders Co, 1983, pp 481–509.

92. Posselt U: Physiology of Occlusion and Rehabilitation. 2nd ed. Philadelphia, FA Davis Co, 1968.

93. Hanamura H, Houston F, Hylander H, Carlsson GE, Haraldson T, Nyman S: Periodontal status and bruxism: A comparative study of patients with periodontal disease and occlusal parafunctions. J Periodontol 1987;58:173–176.

94. Pavone B: Bruxism and its effect on natural teeth. J Prosthet Dent 1985;53:692–696.

95. Posselt U: Treatment of bruxism by bite guards and bite plates. J Can Dent Assoc 1963;29:773–778.

96. Clark GT, Beemsterboer PL, Rugh JD: Nocturnal masseter muscle activity and the symptoms of masticatory dysfunction. J Oral Rhabil 1981;8:279–286.

97. Okeson JP, Kemper JT, Moody PM: A study of the use of occlusion splints in the treatment of acute and chronic patients with craniomandibular disorders. J Prosthet Dent 1982;48:708–712.

98. Laskin DM, Block L: Diagnosis and treatment of myofascial pain dysfunction syndrome. J Prosthet Dent 1986;56:76–84.

99. Carraro JJ, Caffesse RG: Effect of occlusal splints in TMJ symptomology. J Prosthet Dent 1978;40:563–566.

100. Farrar WB: Differentiation of temporomandibular joint dysfunction to simplify treatment. J Prosthet Dent 1972;28:629–636.

101. Farrar WB: Craniomandibular practice: The state of the art; definition and diagnosis. J Craniomand Pract 1982;1:5–12.

102. Clark GT: Treatment of jaw clicking with temporomandibular repositioning: Analysis of 25 cases. J Craniomand Pract 1984;2:263–270.

103. Lundh H, Westesson PL, Kopp S, Tillstrom B: Anterior repositioning splint in the treatment of temporomandibular joints with reciprocal clicking: Comparison with a flat occlusal splint and an untreated control group. Oral Surg Oral Med Oral Pathol 1985;60:131–136.

104. Manns A, Miralles R, Guerrero F: Changes in electrical activity of the postural muscles of the mandible upon varying the

vertical dimension. J Prosthet Dent 1981; 45:438–445.

105. Clark GT, Adler RC: A critical evaluation of occlusal therapy: Occlusal adjustment procedures. J Am Dent Assoc 1985;110: 743–750.

106. Sheikholeslam A, Holmgren K, Riise C: A clinical and electromyographic study of the long-term effects of an occlusal splint on the temporal and masseter muscles in patients with functional disorders and nocturnal bruxism. J Oral Rehabil 1986;13: 137–145.

107. Manns A, Valdivia, Mirralles R, Pena MC: The effect of different occlusal splints on the electromyographic activity of elevator muscles. J Gnathol 1988;7:61–73.

108. Abbott DM, Bush FM: Occlusions altered by removable appliances. J Am Dent 1991; 122:79–81.

109. Fuchs P: The muscular activity of the chewing apparatus during night sleep: An examination of healthy subjects and patients with functional disturbances. J Oral Rehabil 1975;2:35–48.

110. Clark GT, Beemsterboer PL, Solberg WK, Rugh JD: Nocturnal electromyographic evaluation of myofascial pain dysfunction in patients undergoing occlusal splint therapy. J Am Dent Assoc 1979;99:607–611.

111. McNeill C: The optimum temporomandibular joint condyle position in clinical practice. Int J Periodont Rest Dent 1985; 6:52–76.

112. McNeill C: Diagnostic and treatment appliances. In Rhoads J, Rudd KD, Morrow RM (eds) Dental Laboratory Procedures. 2nd ed. St Louis, CV Mosby Co, 1986, pp 428–450.

113. Okeson JP, Moody PM, Kemper JT, Haley J: Evaluation of occlusal splint therapy and relaxation procedures in patients with TMJ disorders. J Am Dent Assoc 1983; 107:420–424.

114. Okeson JP: Management of Temporomandibular Disorders and Occlusion. 2nd ed. St Louis, CV Mosby Co, 1989, pp 413–439.

115. Korioth TWP, Hannam AG: Effect of bilateral asymmetric tooth clenching on load distribution. J Prosthet Dent 1990; 64:62–73.

116. Okeson JP: The effects of hard and soft splints on nocturnal bruxism. J Am Dent Assoc 1987;114:788–791.

117. Shan SC, Yun WH: Influence of an occlusal splint on integrated electromyography of the masseter muscle. J Oral Rehabil 1991;18:253–256.

118. Carr AB, Christensen LV, Donegan SJ, Ziebert GJ: Postural contractible activities of human jaw muscles following use of an occlusal splint. J Oral Rehabil 1991; 18:185–191.

119. Naeije M, Hansson TL: Short term effect of the stabilization appliance in masticatory muscle activity in myogenous craniomandibular disorder patients. J Craniomandib Disord Facial Oral Pain 1991;5:245–250.

120. Dyer EH: Importance of a stable maxillomandibular relation. J Prosthet Dent 1973;30:241–451.

121. Wilkinson T, Hansson TL, McNeill C, Marcel T: A comparison of the success of 24-hour occlusal splint therapy versus nocturnal occlusal splint therapy in reducing craniomandibular disorders. J Craniomandib Disord Facial Oral Pain 1992;6:64–70.

122. Harkins S, Marteney JL, Cueva O, Cueva L: Application of soft occlusal splints in patients suffering from clicking temporomandibular joints. J Craniomand Pract 1988;6:71–76.

123. Ingerslev H: Functional disturbances of the masticatory system in school children. J Dent Child 1983;50(6):446–450.

124. Caswell V: Treatment of anterior displaced meniscus with a flat occlusal splint. J Dent Res 1984;63(special issue):172, abstr 17.

125. Clark GT: TMJ repositioning appliance: A technique for construction, insertion, and adjustment. Cranio 1986;4:37–46.

126. Anderson GC, Schulte JK, Goodking RJ: Comparative study of two treatment methods for internal derangements of the TMJ. J Prosthet Dent 1985;53:392–397.

127. Lundh H, Westesson PL, Jisander S, Eriksson L: Disc repositioning onlays in the treatment of temporomandibular joint disc displacement: Comparison with a flat occlusal splint and no treatment. Oral Surg Oral Med Oral Pathol 1988;66:155–162.

128. Tallents RH, Katzberg RW, Macher DJ, Roberts CA: Use of protrusive splint therapy in anterior disk displacement of the temporomandibular joint: A 1- to 3-year follow-up. J Prosthet Dent 1990;63:336–341.

129. Moloney F, Howard JA: Internal derangements of the temporomandibular joint. III. Anterior repositioning splint therapy. Aust Dent J 1986;31:30–39.

130. Lundh H, Westesson PL: Long-term follow-up after occlusal treatment to correct abnormal temporomandibular joint disc position. Oral Surg Oral Med Oral Pathol 1989;67:2–10.

131. Tallents RH, Katzberg RW, Miller TL, Manzione J, Macher DJ, Roberts C: Arthrographically assisted splint therapy: Painful clicking with a nonreducing meniscus. Oral Surg Oral Med Oral Pathol 1986;61:2–4.

132. Roberts CA, Tallents RH, Katzberg RW, Sanchez-Woodworth RE, Manzione JV, Espeland MA, Hardelman SL: Clinical and arthrographic evaluation of temporomandibular joint sounds. Oral Surg Oral Med Oral Pathol 1986;62:373–376.

133. Ronquillo HI, Guay J, Tallents RH, Katzberg R, Murphy W: Comparison of condyle-fossa relationships with unsuccessful protrusive splint therapy. J Craniomandib Disord Facial Oral Pain 1988;2:178–180.

134. Okeson JP: Long-term treatment of disk-interference disorders of the TMJ with anterior repositioning occlusal splints. J Prosthet Dent 1988;60:611–616.

135. Kirk WS: Magnetic resonance imaging and tomographic evaluation of occlusal appliance treatment for advanced internal derangement of the temporomandibular joint. J Oral Maxillofac Surg 1991;49:9–12.

136. Alanen PJ, Kirveskari PK: Disorders in TMJ research. J Craniomandib Disord Facial Oral Pain 1990;4:223–227.

137. Seligman DA, Pullinger AG: The role of intercuspal occlusal relationships in temporomandibular disorders: A review. J Craniomandib Disord Facial Oral Pain 1991;5:96–106.

138. Seligman DA, Pullinger AG: The role of functional occlusal relationships in temporomandibular disorders: A review. J Craniomandib Disord Facial Oral Pain 1991;5:265–279.

139. Wedel A, Carlsson GE: Factors influencing the outcome of treatment in patients referred to a temporomandibular joint clinic. J Prosthet Dent 1985;54:420–426.

140. Just J, Ayer W, Greene C, Perry H: Treating TM disorders: A survey on diagnosis, etiology and management. J Am Dent Assoc 1991;122:56–60.

141. Pullinger AG, Baldioceda F, Bibb CA: Relationship of TMJ articular soft tissue to underlying bone in young adult condyles. J Dent Res 1990;69:1512–1518.

142. Gausch K: Occlusal therapy of neuromuscular problems in the orofacial region. Int Dent J 1981;31:267–272.

143. Okeson JP: Management of Temporomandibular Disorders and Occlusion. 2nd ed. St Louis, CV Mosby Co, 1989, pp 439–452.

144. Graham GS, Rugh JD: Maxillary splint occlusal guidance patterns and electromyographic activity of the jaw closing muscles. J Prosthet Dent 1988;59:73–77.

145. Rugh JD, Graham GS, Smith JC, Ohrbach RK: Effects of canine versus molar occlusal splint guidance on nocturnal bruxism and craniomandibular symptomatology. J Craniomandib Disord Facial Oral Pain 1989;3:203–210.

146. Minagi S, Akagawa Y, Sato T, Tsuru H: Balancing-side protection: Regulating mechanism of internal derangements of TMJ. J Dent Res 1989;68(special issue): abstr 570.

147. Minagi S, Watanabe H, Sato T, Tsuru H:

The relationship between balancing-side occlusal contact patterns and temporomandibular joint sounds in humans: Proposition of the concept of balancing-side protection. J Craniomandib Disord Facial Oral Pain 1990;4:251–256.

148. Denbo JA: Malocclusion. Dent Clin North Am 1990;34:103–109.

149. Magnusson T, Carlsson GE: Occlusal adjustment in patients with residual or recurrent signs of mandibular dysfunction. J Prosthet Dent 1983;49:706–710.

150. Wennenberg B, Nystrom T, Carlsson GE: Occlusal equilibration and other stomatognathic treatments in patients with mandibular dysfunction and headache. J Prosthet Dent 1988;59:478–483.

151. Schärer P, Stallard E: The effect of occlusal interference on the tooth contact occurrences during mastication. Helv Odont Acta 1966;10:49–56.

152. Clark GT, Mohl ND, Riggs RR: Occlusal adjustment therapy. In Mohl ND, Zarb GA, Carlsson GE, Rugh JD (eds) A Textbook of Occlusion. Chicago, Quintessence Publ Co, 1988, pp 285–303.

153. Goodman P, Greene CS, Laskin DM: Response of patients with myofascial pain-dysfunction to mock equilibration. J Am Dent Assoc 1976;92:755–758.

154. Wise MD: Occlusion and restorative dentistry for the general practitioner. Part I: Preliminary considerations and examination procedures. Br Dent J 1982;152:117–122.

155. Plasmans PJJM, Kuipers L, Vollenbrock HR, Vrijhoef MMA: The occlusal status of molars. J Prosthet Dent 1988;60:500–503.

156. Hannam AG: Optimum occlusal relationships are essential for craniomandibular harmony. Position paper. In Klineberg I, Sessle B (eds) Oro-Facial Pain and Neuromuscular Dysfunction, Mechanisms and Clinical Correlates. Advances in Biosciences. Oxford, Pergamon Press, 1984, pp 167–175.

157. Hylander WL: Mandibular Function and Temporomandibular Joint Loading. Craniofacial Growth Series, No. 16, Ann Arbor, Univ of Michigan, 1985.

158. Faulkner MG, Hatcher DC, Hay A: A three-dimensional investigation of temporomandibular joint loading. J Biomech 1987;20:997–1002.

159. Pekkarinen V, Yli-Urpo A: Helkimo's indices before and after prosthodontic treatment in selected cases. J Oral Rehabil 1987;14:35–42.

160. Perry HT: Diagnosis and treatment of mandibular dysfunction. In Kawamura Y, Dubner R (eds) Oral-Facial Sensory and Motor Function. Chicago, Quintessence Publ Co, 1981, pp 273–282.

161. Perry HT: Occlusal therapy: repositioning. In Laskin D, Greenfield W, Gale E, Rugh J, Neff P, Alling C, Ayer WA (eds) The President's Conference on the Examination, Diagnosis and Management of Temporomandibular Disorders. Chicago, American Dental Association, 1983, pp 155–160.

162. Bradley GR: The effect of splint therapy and orthodontic extrusion on TMJ symptoms. Thesis. St Louis University, St Louis, Missouri, 1989.

163. Greene CS: Orthodontics and the temporomandibular joint. Angle Orthod 1982;52:166–172.

164. Graham GS: Clinical evaluation of temporomandibular disorders. Gen Dent 1983;31:376–379.

165. Pancherz H: The Herbst appliance—its biologic effect and clinical use. Am J Orthod 1985;87:1–20.

166. Nielsen L, Melsen B, Terp S: TMJ function and the effects on the masticatory system on 14–16 year old Danish children in relation to orthodontic treatment. Eur J Orthod 1990;12:254–267.

167. Sadowsky C, Be Gole EA: Longterm status of temporomandibular joint function and functional occlusion after orthodontic treatment. Am J Orthod 1980;78:201–212.

168. Sadowsky C, Polson AM: Temporoman-

dibular disorders and functional occlusion after orthodontic treatments: Results of two long-term studies. Am J Orthod 1984;86:386–390.

169. Gross A, Gale E: Mandibular dysfunction and orthodontic treatment. J Dent Res 1984;63(special issue):354, abstr 1565.

170. Janson M, Hasund A: Function problems in orthodontic patients out of retention. Eur J Orthodont 1981;3:173–179.

171. Gold P: The role of orthodontic treatment and malocclusion in the etiology of mandibular dysfunction. Thesis. University of Manitoba, Canada, 1980.

172. Lieberman MA, Gazit E, Fuchs C, Lilos P: Mandibular dysfunction in 10–18 year old school children as related to morphological malocclusion. J Oral Rehabil 1985;12:215–228.

173. Dahl BJ, Krogstad BS, Ogaard B, Eckersberg T: Signs and symptoms of craniomandibular disorders in two groups of 19-year-old individuals, one treated orthodontically and the other not. Acta Odontol Scand 1988;76:89–93.

174. Sadowsky C, Theisen TA, Sakols EI: Orthodontic treatment and temporomandibular joint sounds—a longitudinal study. Am J Orthod Dentofac Orthop 1991;99:441–447.

175. Eriksson L, Dahlberg G, Westesson P, Petersson A: Changes in TMJ disk position associated with orthognathic surgery. Oral Maxillofac Surg Clin North Am 1990;2:691–698.

176. Dibbets JMH, van der Weele LTh: Extraction, orthodontic treatment, and craniomandibular dysfunction. Am J Orthod Dentofac Orthop 1991;99:210–219.

177. Reynders RM: Orthodontics and temporomandibular disorders: A review of the literature (1966–1988). Am J Orthod Dentofac Orthop 1990;97:463–471.

178. Rendell JK, Norton LA, Gay T: Orthodontic treatment and temporomandibular joint disorders. Am J Orthod Dentofac Orthop 1992;101:84–87.

179. Hirata RH, Heft MW, Hernandez B, King GJ: Longitudinal study of signs of temporomandibular disorders (TMD) in orthodontically treated and nontreated groups. Am J Orthod Dentofac Orthop 1992;101:35–40.

180. Kremenak CR, Kinser DD, Harman HA, Menard CC, Jakoben JR: Orthodontic risk factors for temporomandibular disorders (TMD) I: Premolar extractions. Am J Orthod Dentofac Orthop 1992;101:13–20.

181. Kremenak CR, Kinser DD, Melcher TJ, Wright GR, Harrison SD, Ziaja RR, Harman HA: Orthodontics as a risk factor for temporomandibular disorders (TMD) II. Am J Orthod Dentofac Orthop 1992;101:21–27.

182. Palla S: Untersuchungen zur okklusionsbedingten Distraktion der Kiefergelenke nach orthodontisch indizierter Prämolaren-Extraktion. Thesis. University of Zurich, Zurich, 1972.

183. Kundinger KK, Austin BP, Christensen LV, Donegan SJ, Ferguson DJ: An evaluation of temporomandibular joints and jaw muscles after orthodontic treatment involving premolar extractions. Am J Orthod Dentofac Orthop 1991;100:100–115.

184. Gianelly AA, Hughes HM, Wohlgomuth P, Gildea G: Condylar position and extract treatment. Am J Orthod Dentofac Orthop 1988;93:201–205.

185. Luecke PE, Johnston LE: The effect of maxillary first premolar extraction and incisor retraction on mandibular position: Testing the central dogma of "functional orthodontics." Am J Orthod Dentofac Orthop 1992;101:4–12.

186. Johnston LE, EICO (Orthodontic Study Group of Ohio): Gnathologic assessment of centric slides in post-retention orthodontic patients. J Prosthet Dent 1988;60:712–715.

187. Luecke PE: The effect of maxillary bicuspid extraction treatment of Class II, Division I malocclusion on mandibular position. Thesis, St Louis University, St Louis, Missouri, 1990.

188. Larsson E, Ronnerman A: Mandibular

dysfunction symptoms in orthodontically treated patients ten years after completion of treatment. Eur J Orthodont 1981; 3:89–94.

189. Harmon HA, Jacobsen JR, Juiser DD, Krenenak CR: Premolar extractions for orthodontics as etiologic factors for TMD. J Dent Res 1990;69(special issue): abstr 372.

190. Artun J, Hollender LG, Truelove EL: Relationship between orthodontic treatment, condylar position, and internal derangement in the temporomandibular joint. Am J Orthod Dentofac Orthop 1992;101:48–53.

191. Smith A, Freer TJ: Post-orthodontic occlusal function. Aust Dent J 1989;34:301–309.

192. Egermark I, Thilander B: Craniomandibular disorders with special reference to orthodontic treatment: An evaluation from childhood to adulthood. Am J Orthod Dentofac Orthop 1992;101:28–34.

193. Solberg WK, Seligman DA: Temporomandibular orthopedics: A new vista in orthodontics. In Johnston LA Jr (ed) New Vistas In Orthodontics, Philadelphia, Lea and Ferbiger, 1985, pp 148–183.

194. Athansiou AE, Melsen B, Eriksen J: Concerns, motivation and experiences of orthognathic surgery patients: A retrospective study of 152 patients. Int J Adult Orthod Orthognathic Surg 1989;4:47–55.

195. Ochs M, La Banc JP, Dolwick MF: The diagnosis and management of concomitant dentofacial deformity and temporomandibular disorders. Oral Maxillofac Surg Clin North Am 1990;2:669–690.

196. Proffit WR, White RP: Surgical-orthodontic treatment. Chicago, Mosby Yearbook, 1989, pp 664–665.

197. American Society of Temporomandibular Joint Surgeons: Guidelines for diagnosis and treatment of disorders of the temporomandibular joint and related musculoskeletal disorders. Dallas, 1990.

198. American Association of Oral and Maxillofacial Surgeons. Position paper on TMJ Surgery, 1984.

199. Heffez L, Blaustein D: Diagnostic arthroscopy of the temporomandibular joint. Part I: Normal arthroscopic findings. Oral Surg Oral Med Oral Pathol 1987;64:653–670.

200. Sanders B: Arthroscopic surgery of the temporomandibular joint: Treatment of internal derangement with persistent closed lock. Oral Surg Oral Med Oral Pathol 1986;62:361–372.

201. Sanders B, Buoncristiani R: Diagnostic and surgical arthroscopy of the temporomandibular joint: Clinical experience with 137 procedures over a two year period. J Craniomandib Disord Facial Oral Pain 1987;1:202–213.

202. Forman D: Success with temporomandibular joint arthroscopic surgery. In Controversies in Dentistry. Dent Clin North Am 1990;34:135–140.

203. Clark GT, Moody DG, Sanders B: Arthroscopic treatment of temporomandibular joint locking resulting from disc derangement: Two-year results. J Oral Maxillofac Surg 1991;49:157–164.

204. Blaustein D, Heffez L: Diagnostic arthroscopy to the temporomandibular joint. Part II: Arthroscopic findings of arthrographically diagnosed disc displacement. Oral Surg Oral Med Oral Pathol 1988;65:135–141.

205. American Association of Oral and Maxillofacial Surgeons. Position paper on TMJ Arthroscopy, 1988.

206. Nitzan D, Dolwick MF: An alternative explanation for the genesis of closed-lock symptoms in the internal derangement process. J Oral Maxillofac Surg 1991;49:810–815.

207. Montgomery MT, van Sickels JE, Harms SE: Success of temporomandibular joint arthroscopy in disk displacement with and without reduction. Oral Surg Oral Med Oral Pathol 1991;71:751–759.

208. Moses JJ, Sartoris D, Glass R, Tanaka T, Poker I: The effect of arthroscopic surgi-

cal lysis and lavage of the superior joint space on TMJ disc position and mobility. J Oral Maxillofac Surg 1989;47:674–678.

209. Gabler MJ, Greene CS, Palacios E, Perry HT: Effect of arthroscopic temporomandibular joint surgery on articular disc position. J Craniomandib Disord Facial Oral Pain 1989;3:191–202.

210. Nitzan DW, Dolwick MF, Heft MW: Arthroscopic lavage and lysis of the temporomandibular joint: A change in perspective. J Oral Maxillofac Surg 1990;48:798–801.

211. Perrott DH, Alborzi A, Kaban LB, Helms CA: A prospective evaluation of the effectiveness of temporomandibular joint arthroscopy. J Oral Maxillofac Surg 1990;48:1029–1032.

212. Moses JJ, Topper DC: A functional approach to the treatment of temporomandibular joint internal derangement. J Craniomandib Disord Facial Oral Pain 1991;5:19–27.

213. Nitzan DW, Dolwick MF, Martinez GA: Temporomandibular joint arthrocentesis: A simplified treatment for severe, limited mouth opening. J Oral Maxillofac Surg 1991;49:1163–1167.

214. McCarty WL, Farrar WB: Surgery for internal derangements of the temporomandibular joint. J Prosthet Dent 1979;42:191–196.

215. Tucker MR, Kennedy MC, Jacoway JR: Autogenous auricular cartilage implantation following discectomy in the primate temporomandibular joint. J Oral Maxillofac Surg 1990;48:38–44.

216. Hartog JM, Slavin AB, Kline SN: Reconstruction of the temporomandibular joint with cryo preserved cartilage and freeze-dried dura: A preliminary report. J Oral Maxillofac Surg 1990;48:919–925.

217. Lekkas C, Honee GLJM: The anatomical effects of surgically repositioning the disc in the temporomandibular joint of rats: An experimental study. J Oral Rehabil 1990;17:249–255.

218. Herbosa EG, Rotskoff KS: Composite temporalis pedicle flap as an interpositional graft in temporomandibular joint arthroplasty: A preliminary report. J Oral Maxillofac Surg 1990;48:1049–1056.

219. Pogrel MA, Kaban LB: The role of a temporalis fascia and muscle flap in temporomandibular joint surgery. J Oral Maxillofac Surg 1990;48:14–19.

220. Dolwick MF, Aufdemorte TB: Silicone-induced foreign body reaction and lymphadenopathy after temporomandibular joint arthroplasty. Oral Surg Oral Med Oral Pathol 1985;59:449–452.

221. Westesson PF, Eriksson L, Linstrom C: Destructive lesions of the mandibular condyle following diskectomy with temporary silicone implant. Oral Surg Oral Med Oral Pathol 1987;63:143–150.

222. Heffez L, Mafee MF, Rosenberg H, Langer B: CT evaluation of TMJ disc replacement with a proplast-teflon laminate. J Oral Maxillofac Surg 1987;45:657–665.

223. Florine BL, Gatto DJ, Wade ML, Waite DE: Tomographic evaluation of temporomandibular joints following discoplasty or placement of polytetrafluoroethylene implants. J Oral Maxillofac Surg 1988;48:183–188.

224. Valentine JD: Light and electron microscopic evaluation of proplast II TMJ disc implants. J Oral Maxillofac Surg 1989;47:689–696.

225. Ryan DE: Alloplastic implants in the temporomandibular joint. Oral Maxillofac Clin North Am 1989;1:427–441.

226. Wagner JD, Mosby EL: Assessment of proplast-teflon disc replacements. J Oral Maxillofac Surg 1990;48:1140–1144.

227. Food and Drug Administration: Safety Alerts Department of Health and Human Services. Rockville, Maryland, 1990, 1991.

228. Poswillo DE: Experimental investigation of the effects of intra-articular hydrocortisone and high condylectomy in the mandibular condyle. Oral Surg Oral Med Oral Pathol 1970;30:161–173.

229. Nickerson JW Jr, Veaco NS: Condylot-

omy in surgery of the temporomandibular joint. Oral Maxillofac Surg Clin North Am 1989;1:303–327.

230. Nickerson JW Jr: The role of condylotomy in the management of temporomandibular joint disorders. In Worthington P, Evans J (eds) Controversies in Oral and Maxillofacial Surgery. Philadelphia, Saunders, 1992.

Addendum

Health Care Benefits

Reimbursement

Temporomandibular disorders and orofacial pain are of increasing concern to the general public, clinicians, and researchers. New and improved methods of diagnosis and treatment of TMD now enable patients to benefit from this advanced technology. This surge of interest in the clinical management of these disorders by physicians, dentists, psychologists, physical therapists, and biofeedback therapists has incurred hesitancy among third-party payers who provide health care benefits. There is confusion by these third-party payers as to whether the services should be covered under a patient's medical or dental policy. It is unfortunate that patients who complain of head, neck, and orofacial pains are classified by major medical insurers as suffering from "TMJ" when treatment of the symptoms is provided by a dentist. When the same patient is treated by a physician for the same complaints, the patient is considered to be suffering from a specific medical problem classified according to the symptoms. The designation of a broad, nonspecific category of symptoms classified as "TMJ" perhaps has led carriers to consider benefit coverage for treatment of these symptoms as if they were caused by a single entity with one treatment appropriate in all cases.

Temporomandibular disorders need to be covered under the patient's medical policy on the same basis as are other joint disorders, not under dental or orthodontic policies, regardless of who provides the service, as mandated by the Minnesota Accident and Health Insurance Statutes.[1] Consistent with these statutes, ten other states have legally mandated coverage for nonsurgical and surgical care for TMD on the same basis as for other joints under their medical policies (Kentucky, Maryland, Nevada, New Mexico, North Dakota, Oregon, Tennessee, Texas, Washington, West Virginia).[2] Recently, a federal appeals court in Connecticut upheld a lower court decision ordering a health insurance company to cover a TMD claim under a medical insurance plan.[3] Other state insurance commissioner offices are receiving information on TMD and orofacial pain from dental care councils of state dental associations and the American Dental Association.[4,5] In general, dentists and insurance companies have reacted positively to the use of these guidelines.

Although there continues to be a need for further work in those states with a mandate, progress has been made. As other states attempt to address these same issues, a number of recommendations can be made to enhance patient access to quality and cost-effective care. Changes are best accomplished with a coordinated effort among the university programs, the state dental associations, and health care providers. The state dental associations need to work with medical insurance companies to improve reimbursement for treatment of these disorders and to support legislative efforts to mandate coverage for both surgical and nonsurgical care. Legislation that covers only partial care, such as surgery only, for these problems should be avoided because of the divisive effect that it can have on a patient receiving quality surgical and nonsurgical care. Care should include treatments consistent with those used for other joints and muscles in the body whether administered by physicians, dentists, or other health care providers.

The state dental associations also need to coordinate development of regional practice parameters for the diagnosis, evaluation, and treatment of these disorders. These guidelines should be developed using a broad local representation of academic and private dentists from various specialties and be relatively consistent with national guidelines, eg, the AAOP published guidelines. The guidelines should identify selective treatments and diagnostic tests that have both scientific sup-

port and broad-based agreement on their usefulness, and the criteria for the various diagnostic and treatment modalities need to be periodically reassessed. Guidelines assure credibility to providers and insurance companies, minimize controversy, and ensure access to high-quality, cost-effective care. Insurance companies should be encouraged to use the guidelines as a point of reference for prior authorizations of claims but not to use them literally. Each case needs to be reviewed on an individual basis with use of expert consultants.

Impairment and Disability

The decision on the need for treatment intervention should depend ultimately on three factors—symptom intensity-duration, disability, and progression—rather than on the presence of a symptom. Such an approach would give a legitimate estimate of the problem of TMD in the general population and become a useful goal for health care insurance coverage.[6] The Commission for Evaluation of Pain of the United States Department of Health and Human Services[7] has defined all aspects of pain and has urged that these not be overlooked when evaluating a person for impairment. The Commission describes pain specialists as physicians, psychologists, dentists, and other health professionals who evaluate and treat complex chronic pain problems.[8] Nearly every community, major medical facility, and health education institution has, as a part of its care component, a facility referred to as a "pain center."[9,10]

Of concern is that lack of treatment, inappropriate treatment, or overzealous treatment of a condition with poor results may contribute to or develop into a chronic pain syndrome. Chronic pain behavior in turn can become fixed in the patient's life and can result in the development of dependent relationships, emotional disturbances, physical disabilities, and behavioral and psychosocial disorders. These patients often present with frustrating medical complications that result in unnecessary diagnostic testing, complex treatments, multiple surgical procedures, improper utilization of long-term medications, and dependency on or abuse of the health care system. The past decade has seen an impressive increase in the number of pain management centers or pain clinics that deal with these problems.

Impairment cannot be considered permanent until maximum rehabilitation has been achieved in the attending practitioner's best clinical judgment.[7] It is particularly important to understand the distinction between a patients medical impairment, which is an alteration of health status assessed by medical means, and the patient's disability, which is an alteration of the patient's capacity to meet personal, social, or occupational demands, or to meet statutory or regulatory requirements and is assessed by nonmedical means.[6]

In accordance with the *American Medical Association Guides to the Evaluation of Permanent Impairment*,[11] disability and permanent impairment ratings may be evaluated on either of two conditions: (1) loss of nerve function and (2) conditions that cause interferences in mastication and deglutition (chewing and swallowing). However, these guidelines do not consider limited impairment caused by TMD: (1) the diet is limited to semi-solid or soft foods, 5%; (2) the diet is limited to liquid food, 5% to 10%; (3) ingestion of food requires tube feeding, 10% to 15%.

The issue of TMD impairment and disability merits further evaluation and has been tentatively addressed by an ad hoc insurance committee of the American Academy of Orofacial Pain (AAOP). The proposed AAOP TMD ratings are inclusive of most jaw and facial symptoms except for gross motor weaknesses and sensory loss associated with the trigeminal nerve or disorders of the facial nerve.

Professional Recommendations

Professional Responsibility

The information contained in this document may be useful as a diagnostic and management guide, but the ultimate value of this information for the individual patient depends on the clinician who collects the history, examination, and other diagnostic data and interprets the findings to arrive at a diagnosis. The clinician's most important task and greatest responsibility is to use good clinical judgment to treat the individual patient and avoid approaching all clinical problems as if they were the same. The emphasis should be on conservative therapy that facilitates the musculoskeletal system's natural healing capacity. All dentists are licensed to treat temporomandibular disorders. Each practitioner should assess his or her own knowledge, skill, and ability and should work within his or her own limitations. It is the responsibility of the practitioner to evaluate those patients who have conditions that require greater expertise than they possess and refer them to those who have the capability to provide effective care.

Dentists who choose to manage TMD must use a diagnostic classification stated in terms of established concepts of physiology and pathology such as presented in these guidelines. Even though the proposed biomedical classification system can lead to an appropriate diagnostic label for the condition, clinicians should treat *patients*, not diseases. The weakness of a purely biomedical model is its failure to consider the total patient by ignoring issues of a behavioral, psychologic, or social nature. It is recommended that the clinician consider the biopsychosocial characteristics of the patient's environment when identifying contributing factors in as much as there may be important predisposing, initiating, or perpetuating factors that are not addressed in the biomedical model. Understanding the illness behavior as well as the physical process will result in the more appropriate and successful therapy for the patient.

Proposed treatment should have been proven through controlled research to be both appropriate and effective for the specific disorder(s) being treated.[12] Proposed treatment should have specific value for the disorder as opposed to responses due to nonspecific factors such as placebo effects, positive aspects of the doctor-patient relationship, spontaneous remissions, and overtreatment.[13] This should be reflected in concise and cost-effective treatment plans that avoid use of excessive or untested diagnostic tests, overzealous use of treatments, and open-ended durations of care.

In conclusion, dentistry has accepted the responsibility to provide care for patients with temporomandibular disorders and orofacial pain. Previous experience has shown that we can be successful in treating these patients and gain the respect of patients, other health care providers, and the insurance industry. However, to attain these goals, we need to be aware that the future is dependent on us increasing our scientific knowledge in the area, expanding education in this field, and striving to provide the highest quality and most cost-effective care for our patients.

Educational Responsibility

It is unfortunate that in the past many predoctoral dental educational programs have not trained their students adequately in effective management of orofacial pain and more specifically TMD.[14] Training in the management of chronic pain syndromes in both medical and dental schools has been lacking. Although TMD is a collection of medical conditions, many physicians, including neurologists, orthopedic surgeons, rheumatologists, and otolaryngologists have not been well trained to treat complex chronic pain[15] and often prefer not to treat TMD patients. However, recently a comprehensive core curriculum for professional education in pain was published by The International Association for the Study of Pain Task Force on Professional Education.[16]

Because of their educational concentration and interest in the anatomy, function, and pathophysiology of the jaw and facial structures, dentists will continue to assume the responsibility of diagnosing and treating TMD and orofacial pain. A review of the scientific literature reveals that the majority of basic science and clinical research in this area is accomplished by dentists and is presently proliferating at a rapid rate both in quantity and quality. In light of this, many referrals to dentists and dental clinics specializing in TMD and orofacial pain come from physicians and other health care professionals.

As part of this increasing interest and responsibility, most dental schools have established predoctoral educational programs and some have established postdoctoral residency programs in the evaluation and management of these disorders.[17] Educational guidelines for training programs in dental schools have been established to offer uniformity in clinical practice based on generally accepted practice parameters.[18–21]

A majority of practicing dentists treating TMD patients, however, have not had formal training or credentialing in the diagnosis and management of TMD and orofacial pain. And, unfortunately, continuing education programs, which proliferated over the last decade, disseminated TMD information with a wide range of scientific integrity and inconsistency in terminology, diagnostic criteria, and management protocol.[22] The establishment of definitive guidelines for the presentation of continuing education in TMD has been difficult due to the wide variety of course lengths, course objectives, faculty, and location of courses. Therefore, the responsibility for training dentists into the next century in this complex and important area must, in large part, be met by more effective continuing education programs. The overall goal should be an effort to organize, coordinate, and unify philosophies and clinical techniques. This attempt should establish scientifically based programs that include the integration and correlation of related basic and clinical sciences and dental techniques.[23]

Course content should be scientifically valid and presented in an academically honest context.[24] Participants have the right to expect information to be accurate and documentable in refereed journals. This is not to say that new or scientifically undocumented information should never be presented, but it should be identified as such. Clinical programs should be multidisciplinary, when appropriate, and based on an acceptable diagnostic classification system. Professional excellence is dependent on the quality of the education of health care providers. Continuing education facilities must attempt to integrate their programs with degree- or credential-granting institutions in all the health sciences. The ultimate goal of this educational process is to permit dentists to provide the best possible care for their patients.

Academy Responsibility

This document should be referenced in the time frame in which it has been written. The American Academy of Orofacial Pain anticipates the need to continually revise these published guidelines with input from all who support or take exception to the information provided. While it is the hope of the Academy that these practice guidelines will improve the quality of patient care,[25] this is not a standard of care document. The standard of care must be established locally. However, it is hoped that it will serve as a nucleus for discussions on the standard of care by all interested parties. We are reluctant to label this as a "state of the art" document because the "state of the art" is in a constant state of flux due to the fact that the field is ever changing for the benefit of all.

References

1. Minnesota Accident and Health Insurance Statutes Dental Procedures. Chap 62A.043, 1987(Suppl).

2. American Dental Association: Department of State Government Affairs. J Am Dent Assoc 1991;122:83–84.

3. Spaeth D: Court orders insurer to pay TMJ claim. Am Dent Assoc News 1991;22:9.

4. California Dental Association Council on Dental Care: Guidelines for the assessment of clinical quality and professional performance: TMJ and MPD Guidelines. California Dental Association, 1989.

5. American Dental Association, Council on Dental Care Programs: Prepayment plan benefits for temporomandibular joint dis-

orders. J Am Dent Assoc 1982;105:485–488.

6. Pullinger AG, Moneiro AA: Functional impairment in TMJ patient and nonpatient groups according to a disability index and symptom profile. J Craniomand Pract 1988; 6:156–165.

7. Commission for Evaluation of Pain: United States Department of Health and Human Services, Social Security Administration, Office of Disability, March 1984, p 134.

8. Phillips DJ, Walters PJ, Rogal OJ, Stack BC, Weiner LB, Klemons IM: Recommended guide to the evaluation of permanent impairment of the temporomandibular joint. J Craniomand Pract 1989;7:13–17.

9. International Association for the Study of Pain: Task force on guidelines for disenable characteristics for pain treatment facilities. IASP, Seattle, Washington, 1990.

10. Brena SF, Sanders SH: The business of pain management programs: How to plan and successfully operate a pain management facility. Am Pain Soc Bull 191;1:4–6.

11. American Medical Association: Guides to the Evaluation of Permanent Impairment. 2nd ed. Chicago, American Medical Association, 1984.

12. Mohl ND, Ohrbach R: The dilemma of scientific knowledge versus clinical management of temporomandibular disorders. J Prosthet Dent 1992;67:113–120.

13. Greene CS: A critique of non-conventional treatment concepts and procedures for TM Disorders. In Laskin D, Greenfield W, Gale E, Rugh J, Neff P, Alling C, Ayer WF (eds) The President's Conference on the Examination, Diagnosis and Management of Temporomandibular Disorders. Am Dent Assoc, 1983, pp 177–181.

14. McNeill C, Mohl ND, Rugh JD, Tanaka TT: Temporomandibular disorders: Diagnosis, management, education, and research. J Am Dent Assoc 1990;120:253–263.

15. Pilowsky I: An outline curriculum on pain for medical schools. Pain 1988;33:1–2.

16. Fields HL: Core curriculum for professional education in pain. Task force on professional education. International Association for the Study of Pain, Seattle, IASP Publ, 1991.

17. Gonty AA: Teaching a comprehensive orofacial pain course in the dental curriculum. J Dent Educ 1990;54:319–322.

18. Attanasio R, Mohl ND: Curriculum guidelines for the development of predoctoral programs in temporomandibular disorders. J Dent Educ 1992;56:646–649.

19. Attanasio R, Mohl ND: Curriculum guidelines for the development of postdoctoral programs in temporomandibular disorders and orofacial pain. J Dent Educ 1992;56: 650–658.

20. Attanasio R, Mohl ND: Suggested curriculum guidelines for the development of predoctoral programs in TMD and orofacial pain. J Craniomandib Disord Facial Oral Pain 1992;6:113–116.

21. Attanasio R, Mohl ND: Suggested curriculum guidelines for the development of postdoctoral programs in TMD and orofacial pain. J Craniomandib Disord Facial Oral Pain 1992;6:126–134.

22. Rugh JD, Solberg WK: Oral health status in the United States temporomandibular disorders. J Dent Educ 1985;49:398–405.

23. McNeill C, Falace D, Attanasio R: Continuing education for TMD and orofacial pain: A philosophical overview. J Craniomandib Disord Facial Oral Pain 1992;6: 135–136.

24. Association of University TMD Orofacial Pain Centers, Planning Session, San Francisco, American Association of Dental Research Meeting, 1989.

25. Crall JJ: The role of health services research in developing practice policy: Development of practice guidelines. J Dent Educ 1990;54:693–694.

Glossary

A

abrasion of teeth Pathologic wearing away of teeth from mastication or bruxism in contrast to chemical erosion.

abscess Localized collection of pus within tissues or preformed cavities.

acoustic meatus External cartilaginous and internal bony auditory canal.

acoustic neuroma Benign tumor within the auditory canal arising from the eighth cranial (acoustic) nerve [CN VIII].

acquired disorder Postnatal aberration, change, or disturbance of normal development or condition that relates to the individual and is not bound to hereditary transmission from parents to offspring.

acromegaly Chronic metabolic condition characterized by a gradual and marked elongation and enlargement of bones of the face, jaws, and extremities, accompanied by enlargement of the lips and thickening of the soft tissues of the face, which afflicts middle-aged persons and is caused by overproduction of growth hormone.

activation of muscles Energy release in muscle caused by the passage of molecules through membranes that takes the system from its normal resting state to one of muscle contraction.

active mandibular opening Mandibular range of motion achieved by motion imparted by voluntary contraction of the controlling muscles and relaxation of antagonist muscles.

active resistive stretch Motion voluntarily imparted against resistance of muscle, tendons, capsule, or intra-articular structures.

acupuncture Traditional Chinese practice of inserting needles into specific points along the "meridians" of the body to induce anesthesia, for alleviating pain or for prevention. There is experimental evidence that the procedure produces an analgesic effect because it causes the release of enkephalin, a naturally occurring endorphin that has opiatelike effects.

acute [*ant*: **chronic**] Having rapid onset, severe symptoms, or short course.

acute malocclusion Malocclusion with sudden onset, related to joint pain, inflammation, and/or protective muscle splinting.

acute pain Unpleasant sensation with duration of pain related to the normal healing time of the initiating or causal factors.

adaptive capacity [*syn*: **adaptive potential, adaptive response**] Relative ability to adjust to a change in the environment. More specifically, the correlation between the change in structure and the change in function of tissues dependent upon the conditions of their local environment.

adenocarcinoma Malignant adenoma arising from the epithelium of a glandular organ.

adenoma Neoplasm arising from glandular epithelium.

adenopathy Swelling or enlargement of any gland, especially a lymph node.

adenosine triphosphate [**ATP**] Enzyme found in muscle cells, responsible for producing energy.

adherence Binding or sticking of opposing surfaces.

adhesion Molecular attraction between two surfaces in contact. The abnormal joining or union of adjacent structures, or any band that connects them, as may occur in an inflammatory process or as the result of injury.

capsular adhesions Fibrosis of the capsular structures.

extracapsular adhesion Fibrosis of tissue adjacent to capsule such as muscles or ligaments, ie, collateral ligament fibrous, adhesion of coronoid process and temporalis muscle, or other muscle of mastication adhering to adjacent cranial structures.

intracapsular adhesions Fibrous bands or adhesions between intra-articular surfaces, including the surrounding capsule.

adhesiotomy Surgical separation of adhesions.

adhesive capsulitis Adhesions between capsule/disc/fossa/condyle resulting in reduced joint space volume and causing restricted translation or rotation. In the TMJ the disc position may be normal but with reduced mobility. Diagnosis determined with arthrography.

adjunctive therapy An addition to the principal procedure or primary course of therapy.

affect In psychology, the emotional reactions associated with an experience.

afferent neural pathway Nerve impulses transmitted from the periphery toward the central nervous system.

agenesis Failure of development of a part in the absolute sense. Nonappearance of the primordium in the embryo.

agonist [*ant*: **antagonist**] Muscle principally responsible for a particular movement.

algometer Instrument for measuring degree of sensitivity to pressure pain.

allodynia Pain that occurs without noxious stimulus at the anatomic site of the pain.

alloplastic implant Nonbiologic material implanted surgically to augment or replace tissue.

alveolar Pertaining to a tooth socket, supporting bone, and associated connective tissue.

ameloblastoma Tumor of the jaw arising from the enamel organ, of low grade malignancy.

analgesia Absence of normal sense of pain.

analgesic Agent that alleviates or reduces pain without loss of consciousness.

anamnestic Pertaining to past medical history.

anatomic Pertaining to morphology, the structure of an organism.

anesthesia Partial or complete loss of sensation with or without loss of consciousness.

anesthesia dolorosa [*syn*: **postsurgical neuralgia**] Loss of sensation of a part but with paradoxical pain.

aneurysm Localized, abnormal dilation of a blood vessel, usually an artery.

Angle's classification of malocclusion Classification of dental malocclusion based on the relationship of the maxillary and mandibular molar and incisor teeth.

Class I Minor dental irregularities but a correct anteroposterior relationship of the maxillary to the mandibular teeth.

Class II Mandible and its teeth are in a posterior or retruded relationship to the maxillary teeth.

division 1 Maxillary anterior teeth have a normal or excessive forward inclination, often with excessive horizontal overjet.

division 2 Maxillary incisors are upright or inclined backward, often with an excessive overbite.

Class III Mandible and its teeth are positioned too far forward in relationship to the maxilla.

anhydrosis Absence of or reduced sweating.

ankylosing spondylitis Ossification of ligaments that results in bony encasement of the joint, primarily in spine, onset suggestive of rheumatoid arthritis with gradual progressive movement restriction of the affected joints. Represents 15% of cases of arthritis that begin before the age of 16 years, with HLA B27 antigen almost always found. More common in men with onset most often between 9 to 12 years of age.

ankylosis Immobility or fixation of a joint as a result of fibrous or bony union that may be congenital or the result of disease, trauma or surgery.

bony ankylosis [*syn:* **synostosis**] Imaging evidence of reduced joint space with osseous union and lack of translatory movement.

fibrous ankylosis [*syn:* **pseudoankylosis**] Fibrous adhesions and capsular fibrosis.

anorexia Diminished appetite, aversion to food.

anorexia nervosa Personality disorder usually occurring in young women, characterized by extreme aversion to food and resulting in extreme weight loss and amenorrhea.

antagonist [*ant:* **agonist**] Muscle whose function is opposite the agonist or prime mover.

antegonial notching Depression or concavity at the inferior aspect of the body of the mandible at the junction with ramus, near the insertion of the masseter muscle.

anterior [*ant:* **posterior**] Toward the front.

anterior positioning appliance Intraoral device that guides the mandible to a position forward of maximum intercuspation.

antinuclear antibody [**ANA**] Anti-DNA antibody of serum lupus erythematosus and other connective tissue disorders.

antipyretic Fever-reducing medication.

anxiety Feeling of apprehension, uncertainty, or dread of a future threat or danger, accompanied by tension or uneasiness.

anxiety disorder [*syn:* **panic disorder**] Chronic and persistent apprehension manifested by autonomic hyperactivity such as sweating, dizziness, heart palpitations, musculoskeletal hyperactivity, and irritability.

aplasia Incomplete or arrested development of a structure due to failure of normal development of the embryonic primordium.

apnea Temporary cessation of breathing.

aponeurosis Flat, fibrous sheath of connective tissue that attaches muscle to bone or other tissue.

appliance Device or prosthesis to provide or facilitate a particular function or therapy.

arch length discrepancy Inadequate dental arch circumference to accommodate the mesial to distal dimensions or the interproximal contact points of the natural teeth.

arteriovenous malformation Altered morphology, weakening or distension of an artery or vein.

arteritis Inflammation of an artery, usually of the intima or internal layers.

arthralgia Pain in and around a joint.

arthritis [*pl.,* **arthritides**] Inflammation of a joint and peri-articular tissues, usually accompanied by pain.

arthritis deformans [*unfavorable term*] See **arthrosis**.

arthrocentesis Puncture of a joint space by using a needle, followed by removal of fluid.

arthrodial Gliding joint movement.

arthrogram Visualization of a joint by radiography following injection of a radiopaque contrast agent into the joint space to determine the location and integrity of intra-articular soft tissue structures including disc position, soft tissue contours, presence of perforations, joint motion, intra-articular free bodies, and adhesive capsulitis.

single contrast Injection of a radiopaque contrast agent.

double contrast Injection of a small amount of radiopaque contrast agent followed by inflation of the joint with air.

single space Injection of a radiopaque contrast agent into either the upper or the lower synovial bursa of the TMJ.

double space Injection of a radiopaque contrast agent into both the upper and lower synovial bursa of the TMJ.

arthrogryposis Fixation of a joint in a flexed or contracted position that may be related to innervation, muscles, or connective tissue.

arthrokinematics See **arthrokinetics**.

arthokinetics [*syn:* **arthrokinematics**] Joint motion.

depression of mandible Downward movement of the mandible.

distraction of mandible Separation of surfaces of the temporomandibular joint by extension without injury or dislocation of the parts.

elevation of mandible Upward movement of the mandible.

lateral excursion of mandible Eccentric movement by condylar translation to the contralateral side.

laterotrusion of mandible Movement of the mandible away from the median or toward the side.

mediotrusion of mandible Movement of the mandible toward the median or center.

protrusion of mandible Eccentric movement with bilateral forward condylar translation.

retrusion of mandible Bilateral condylar translation in a posterior direction.

arthropathy Any disease or disorder that affects a joint.

arthroplasty Surgical repair or plastic reconstruction of a joint.

arthroscopy Direct visualization of a joint with an endoscope.

arthrosis Trophic degeneration of a joint.

arthrotomography Tomographic radiographs taken following the injection of radiopaque contrast medium into a joint.

arthrotomy Surgical incision of a joint.

articular Pertaining to a joint.

articular capsule Fibrous connective envelope of tissue that surrounds a synovial joint.

articular disc See **disc**.

articulate In dentistry, the state of the teeth being brought together into occlusion.

articulation Union between two or more bones.

articulator Mechanical device for attachment of dental casts that allows movement of the casts into various eccentric relationships.

asymmetry Lack of symmetry, unequal in size, shape, movement, or function.

ataxia Impaired ability to coordinate movement, neuromuscular dysfunction.

attrition Wearing away by friction or rubbing. A wearing away of teeth in the normal course of use.

attrition bruxism Tooth grinding with frictional wear of opposing teeth in excursive movements, in contrast to tooth clenching.

atypical facial pain Continuous, unilateral, deep, aching pain, sometimes with a burning component. Unfavorable term as the underlying cause for the symptoms may just not have been discovered, and the symptom complex should be referred to as facial pain of unknown origin.

atypical odontalgia [*unfavorable term*] See **idiopathic odontalgia**.

atrophy [*ant:* **hypertrophy**] Progressive decline or wasting away of tissue, eg, bone resorption, muscle disuse atrophy.

auditory nerve Sensory cranial nerve (CN VIII) with cochlear (hearing) and vestibular (equilibrium) fibers.

aura Subjective sensation or phenomenon that precedes and marks the onset of a paroxysmal attack.

auricle [*syn:* **pinna**] Portion of the external ear outside the head that connects to the external auditory meatus, the portion of the external ear contained within the head.

auriculotemporal nerve Sensory branch of the mandibular division of the trigeminal nerve. Innervates the external acoustic meatus, the lateral aspect of the temporomandibular joint capsule, the parotid sheath, and the skin of the auricle.

auriculotemporal neuralgia Paroxysmal pain with refractory periods of the auriculotemporal branch of the trigeminal nerve.

auscultation Listening for sounds within the body, a diagnostic method.

autogenous graft Graft transferred from one part of a patient's body to another.

autoimmune disorder Disease in which the body produces a disordered immunologic response against itself, causing tissue injury, eg, rheumatoid arthritis, scleroderma.

autonomic nervous system Regulates involuntary vital functions including cardiac muscle, smooth muscle, and glands, including salivary, sweat, and gastric glands. Comprised of sympathetic and parasympathetic divisions.

avascular Lacking in blood vessels or having a poor blood supply.

avascular necrosis [AVN] Bone infarction not associated with asepsis but with circulatory impairment (vascular occlusion) leading to bone necrosis and collapse of joint surface into underlying infarction.

B

balancing occlusal contact [*unfavorable term*] See **nonworking occlusal contact**.

behavior Actions or reactions under specific circumstance.

behavior modification Psychotherapy that attempts to modify observable patterns of behavior by the substitution of a new response to a given stimulus.

benign Mild, nonprogressive character of an illness that may disturb function without endangering the life of the individual, nonmalignant character of a tumor.

benign masseteric hypertrophy Nonmalignant increase in size or bulk of masseter muscles of unknown etiology, usually bilateral.

bilaminar zone [*unfavorable term*] See **retrodiscal tissue**.

bilateral [*ant*: **unilateral**] Pertaining to or having two sides.

biofeedback training Utilizing equipment to feed back a visual or auditory representation of a measured physiologic activity or autonomic function, used in therapy to voluntarily modify physiologic activity or autonomic function.

biomechanical Action of intrinsic or extrinsic forces on the body, in particular the locomotor system.

block anesthesia Regional anesthesia resulting from nerve block by injecting into or near a nerve trunk.

border movements Movements of the mandible at the boundary or margin of the envelope of movement. Determined by the joint anatomy, joint capsule, ligaments, and associated muscles.

bracing [*syn*: **clenching**] Static, prolonged position of the mandible maintained by masticatory and tongue muscle activity, not necessarily involving contact of the teeth.

bradykinin Plasma kinin that is a potent vasodilator and incites pain.

brain stem Connects cerebral hemispheres with the spinal cord, comprised of the medulla oblongata, pons, and the midbrain.

bruxism Diurnal or nocturnal parafunctional activity including clenching, bracing, gnashing, and grinding of the teeth. In absence of subjective awareness, can be diagnosed from presence of clear wear facets that are not generated by masticatory function.

bruxism appliance Intraoral device for controlling or reducing bruxism activity and associated discomfort or damage to the dentition.

bulimia Craving for food, often resulting in episodes of continuous, binge eating followed by periods of depression and self-deprivation.

bulimia nervosa Personality disorder usually seen in young women, a variety of anorexia nervosa with bouts of overeating followed by intentional, self-induced vomiting. Characterized by chemical erosion of teeth from stomach acids and may result in bilateral enlargement of the parotid glands.

bursa Sac-like cavity found in connective tissue at places where friction would otherwise develop. Lined with synovial membrane and filled with viscous synovial fluid.

bursitis Inflammation of a bursa.

C

calcium pyrophosphate dihydrate crystals Present in synovial fluid of joint affected by active attack of gout.

capsulitis Inflammatory response of capsule and associated capsular ligament and disc attachments in response to mechanical irritation or systemic disease.

carotid artery Principal artery of the neck, the paired common carotid, divides at the upper border of the thyroid cartilage into the external and internal carotid arteries.

carotodynia Pain in the distribution of the branches of the external carotid artery, usually related to pressure on the artery.

cast In dentistry, a model or representation of the teeth and supporting bone, usually made of stone or plaster.

caudal [*syn*: **inferior**, *ant*: **cephalic**] Inferior, toward the tail.

causalgia [*syn*: **reflex sympathetic dystrophy**] Deafferentation pain initiated by trauma or surgical procedure.

central nervous system [CNS] Brain and spinal cord, processes information to and from the peripheral nervous system and is the network of coordination and control of the entire body.

centric occlusion [CO] [*syn*: **maximum intercuspal position**] That position of the mandible relative to the maxilla where the greatest degree of tooth contact is achieved on articulation of the teeth.

centric relation [CR] See **centric relation occlusion**.

centric relation occlusion [CRO] [*syn*: **centric relation, retruded contact position**] Position of the mandible relative to the maxilla, defined when normal joint anatomy exists, such that on pure rotation (hinge closure) the mandibular condyle is functioning in its most physiologic position. Determined at the point of initial tooth contact on this arc of physiologic closure, not necessarily coincident with centric occlusion.

cephalic [*syn*: **rostral**, *ant*: **caudal**] Toward the head, structure of the head.

cephalgia [*syn*: **headache**] Pain or ache in the head.

cephalogram Radiogram of the head.

cerebral palsy Motor function disorder caused by a permanent, nonprogressive brain defect or lesion present at birth or shortly thereafter. Deep tendon reflexes are exaggerated, fingers are often spastic, and speech may be slurred.

cervical Pertaining to the neck.

cervicalgia Pain of the structures of the neck, may be referred pain from noncervical origin.

cervicogenic Originating in the structures of the neck.

chief complaint [CC] Purpose of patient's visit, most bothersome, most desired to be changed.

chondritis Inflammation of cartilage.

chondroblastoma Benign tumor, derived from precursors of cartilage cells, that may contain scattered areas of calcification and necrosis.

chondroma Benign cartilaginous tumor.

chondromalacia Softening of cartilage that may be accompanied by swelling, pain, and degeneration.

chondrosarcoma Malignant tumor of cartilaginous cells or their precursors that may contain nodules of calcified hyaline cartilage.

chronic [*ant*: **acute**] Developing slowly and persisting for a long time.

chronic pain Enduring and relatively constant condition that has become a component of the patients' daily routine. May have associated unpleasant sensory, perceptual, and emotional experiences with associated behavioral and psychosocial responses. Persistent pain beyond 6 months or the normal time for healing of an acute injury or pain that persists when other aspects of disorder-disease have resolved.

chronic paroxysmal hemicrania Rare form of headache centered around the eye and radiating to the cheek or temple with attacks lasting 5 to 60 minutes with 4 to 12 attacks per day for years without remission. Like cluster headache, may have associated conjunctival congestion and clear nasal discharge, with the headache consistently remaining on the same side.

claudication Pain in muscle resulting from inadequate blood supply.

clenching [*syn*: **bracing**] Exertion of masticatory force, primarily of the elevator muscles, in static occlusal relationship that is not associated with normal functions such as biting, chewing, swallowing, or speech. May be diurnal or nocturnal and the patient may not be aware of the muscle activity.

clicking joint noise Distinct snapping or popping sound emanating from the TMJ during joint movement or with joint compression.

cluster headache [*syn*: **Horton's syndrome, histamine cephalgia**] Severe unilateral head and face pain, often accompanied by involuntary lacrimation, with localized extracranial vasodilatation in the periorbital region contributing to the pain and conjunctival congestion. The paroxysmal pain occurs in bouts or clusters, sometimes with clockwork regularity, with the attacks usually occurring during the night, lasting 30 to 120 minutes.

cognitive behavioral therapy Therapy focused on changing attitudes, perceptions, and patterns of thinking.

collateral ligament Supportive ligament on the lateral aspect of the temporomandibular joint capsule.

compression of joint Pressing together of joint surfaces.

computed tomography [**CT**] Tomographic method that employs a narrowly collimated radiographic beam that passes through the body and is recorded by an array of scintillation detectors. The computer calculates tissue absorption, demonstrating the densities of various structure.

condyle Rounded, articular end of a bone.

condylar fracture Fracture of the head or neck of the mandibular condyle that may be intracapsular or extracapsular and may be displaced or nondisplaced.

condylectomy Surgical removal of a portion of the superior mandibular condylar head.

condyloid Pertaining to the condylar process.

condylotomy [*syn*: **subcondylar osteotomy**] Surgical sectioning of the condylar neck without removal or recontouring of the condyle.

condylysis [*syn*: **condylolysis**] Resorption or dissolution of condyle.

congenital disorder Developmental disorder present at birth.

conjunctiva Mucous membrane covering the anterior surface of the eyeball and lining the eyelids.

conjunctival injection Dilation of the vascularature of the conjunctiva.

connective tissue Tissue of mesodermal origin that supports and connects other tissues and includes elastic or collagenous fibrous connective tissue, bone, and cartilage. Connective tissues are highly vascular with the exception of cartilage.

connective tissue disorder [*syn*: **mixed connective tissue disease, collagen disease**] Group of diseases of connective tissue that share common anatomic and pathologic features. The etiology of these diseases is unknown and they are grouped on the basis of common clinical signs and symptoms.

continuous passive motion [**CPM**] Cyclic motion imparted to a body part by another individual or machine that moves an articulation through a determined range of motion.

contracture Abnormal, usually permanent, condition of a joint caused by the loss of the normal elasticity of the skin or connective tissue surrounding a joint or by atrophy and shortening of the muscles.

contraction Shortening, tightening, or reduction in size or length of a muscle fiber.

contralateral [*ant*: **ipsilateral**] Originating in or affecting the opposite side.

contrast medium Radiopaque material injected prior to imaging examination that renders certain tissues or spaces opaque.

contributing factor Condition or action that contributes to the occurrence of or aggravation of a disease or disorder.

contusion of joint Traumatic condition not sufficient to cause condylar fracture, characterized by acute synovitis, effusion, and possible hemarthrosis.

conversion disorder Repressed emotional conflicts that are converted into sensory, motor, or visceral symptoms with no underlying organic cause. The conversion reaction often becomes evident through a hysterical manifestation of symptoms resembling those of an organic disease.

coping mechanisms Cognitive and behavioral efforts to manage specific tasks, problems, or situations.

coronal [*syn:* **frontal**] Vertical plane, perpendicular to sagittal plane, dividing the body into front to back portions.

coronoid hyperplasia Benign overgrowth of the coronoid process of the mandible that may result in limited opening.

coronoid process Process on the anterosuperior surface of the mandibular ramus that serves as the attachment of the temporalis muscle.

coronoid process impingement Hyperplastic growth disturbance resulting in progressive, gradual restriction of mouth opening caused by obstruction of the hyperplastic coronoid process by the zygomatic process. Restriction is more pronounced if opening is attempted from a protruded or translatory condylar position. Relative impingement can also occur without hyperplasia of coronoid when there has been shortening of the condylar head with superior positioning of the condylar articular surface.

corrected cephalometric tomography Tomography of structures of the head, in particular the condyle of the mandible, with the radiographic section oriented to the precise location and angulation of the structure of interest.

Costen's syndrome Syndrome of dizziness, tinnitus, earache, stuffiness of the ear, dry mouth, burning in the tongue and throat, sinus pain, and headaches that an otolaryngologist in 1934 attributed to overclosure of the bite and posterior displacement of the mandibular condyle.

cranial [*syn:* **cephalic, superior**] In the direction of the head, pertaining to the structures of the head.

cranial arteritis [*syn:* **giant cell arteritis**] Condition characterized by fever, anorexia, loss of weight, leucocytosis, tenderness over the scalp and along facial and temporal arteries, headache, and jaw claudication. May lead to blindness. Age related onset, uncommon before the age of 60 years. Cranial manifestation of giant cell arteritis.

cranial nerves [**CN**] Twelve pairs of nerves that have their origin in the brain.

craniocervical Relating to both the cranium and the neck.

craniofacial Relating to both the face and the cranium.

craniomandibular Paired articulation of the mandible to the cranium.

craniomandibular disorder [**CMD**] [*unfavorable term*] See **temporomandibular disorder**.

cranium Skull or bones of the head that encase the brain.

crepitation [*syn:* **grating, crepitus**] Noise or vibration produced by rubbing bone or irregular cartilage surfaces together, as found with arthrosis.

crossbite Condition in which normal labiolingual or buccolingual relationship between the maxillary and mandibular teeth is reversed.

cutaneous Relating to the skin.

D

deafferentation pain Pain perceived in a localized area resulting from the loss or disruption of sensory nerve fibers.

debridement Excision of devitalized tissue and foreign matter from a diseased area or wound.

decompression of a joint Removal or release of pressure.

deflection on mandibular opening Eccentric displacement of mandible on opening, away from a centered mandibular midline path, without correction to midline position on full opening.

degeneration Tissue deterioration with soft tissue, cartilage, and bone converted into or replaced by tissue of inferior quality. Failure of articulation to adapt to loading forces, resulting in impaired function.

deglutition The act of swallowing.

delayed onset muscle soreness Pain caused by intermittent overuse, resulting in interstitial inflammation.

delta sleep Nonrapid eye movement, Stage IV sleep.

demyelination Loss of myelin from the sheath of a nerve.

dental Pertaining to a tooth or teeth.

dentition Arrangement of the natural teeth in the dental arch.

depression of mandible Downward movement; a component of normal mandibular opening.

depressive state Psychiatric mood disorder.

derangement A disturbed arrangement; a mechanical disorder.

developmental disorder See **acquired disorder, congenital disorder**.

deviation in form Irregularities or aberrations in the form of intracapsular, soft, and hard articular tissue.

deviation on mandibular opening Eccentric displacement of mandible on opening, away from centered mandibular midline path, with correction to midline position on full opening.

diagnosis Determining the nature of a disease from a study of the signs and symptoms.

differential diagnosis Differentiation of two or more diseases with similar symptoms to determine which is the correct diagnosis.

digingylmoarthroidal Paired joint that is both a hinged (ginglymoid) and a gliding (arthrodial) joint.

disability Alteration of the patient's capacity to meet personal or social demands or occupational tasks. Failure to meet statutory or regulatory requirements. Assessed by nonphysical measures such as social adjustment or psychological assessment.

disc [*syn: **articular disc, intra-articular disc**] Intra-articular, plate-like fibrocartilaginous structure in the TMJ consisting of an anterior band, intermediate zone, and posterior band.

disc derangement See **internal derangement**.

disc displacement Abnormal position of the intra-articular disc relative to the mandibular condyle and the temporal fossa.

reducing Condyle re-establishes a normal anatomic relationship with the disc during condylar translation or rotation.

nonreducing Condyle fails to re-establish a normal anatomic relationship with the disc during condylar translation or rotation.

disc interference disorder See **internal derangement**.

discal repositioning surgery Arthrotomy with intent of re-establishing normal disc-to-condyle anatomic relationship.

discectomy [*syn: meniscectomy*] Arthrotomy with removal of intra-articular disc.

disclusion [*syn: disocclusion*] Separation of mandible from maxilla in excursive movements through tooth-guided contact.

discoplasty Correction or improvement in the contour or position of a disc.

disease Illness, sickness, body function disorder, or pathologic alterations characterized by identifiable group of signs and symptoms.

disk [*unfavorable term*] See **disc**.

dislocation of condyle Anterior displacement of mandibular condyle away from the temporal component, lacking contact with normal articulating surface but located within the joint capsule.

disorder Disturbance of function, structure, or both.

displacement Removal from the normal or usual position or place.

distal [*ant: **proximal**] Away from the origin.

distraction of the condyle Separation or downward movement of the condylar head from the normal articular contact zone.

diurnal [*ant: **nocturnal**] Pertaining to or occurring in the daylight hours.

dizziness Sensation of faintness or inability to maintain normal balance, sometimes with associated mental confusion, nausea, and weakness.

Doppler effect The apparent change in the frequency of a wave resulting from relative motion of the source and the receiver.

Doppler ultrasonography The application of the Doppler effect to ultrasonic scanning with ultrasound echoes converted to (amplified) sound or graphic waves.

dysarthrosis Deformity or malformation of a joint whereby there is impairment of joint motion.

dyscrasia Morbid condition referring to an imbalance of the component parts.

dysesthesia Disagreeable or impaired (abnormal) sensation.

dysfunction Collective term for signs and symptoms of abnormal or altered function.

dyskinesia Motor function disorder with impairment of voluntary movement, characterized by spontaneous, imprecise, involuntary, irregular movements with stereotype patterns. May involve grimacing, muscle tremors, and sudden twitches as occur from the adverse effect of phenothiazine derivative medications.

dysostosis Abnormal condition characterized by defective ossification, especially defects in the ossification of fetal cartilages.

dysphoria Disquiet, restlessness, malaise.

dysplasia Pathologic abnormality of development or replacement of cells with alteration in the size, shape, and organization.

dystonia Abnormal tonicity, usually in reference to muscle tissue, that may result in altered movement and posture.

focal dystonia Localized dystonia characterized by momentary sustained contracture of involved muscles.

dystrophy Developmental change in muscles resulting from defective nutrition, not involving the central nervous system, with fatty degeneration and increased size but decreased strength.

E

eccentric Jaw relation or position that is peripheral or away from a centered or centric jaw position.

edema Abnormal accumulation of fluid in cells, tissue, or cavities.

efferent neural pathway Neural impulse transmitted away from the central nervous system.

efficacy Maximum ability of a drug or treatment to produce a result, regardless of dosage or frequency.

effusion Escape of fluid from blood vessels or lymphatics, usually into a body cavity or tissue.

Ehlers-Danlos syndrome Autosomal dominant inherited disorder of dermal collagen, lax joints, and skin elasticity.

elastic tissue Connective tissue composed of approximately 30% elastin, a yellow fibrous mucoprotein.

electrogalvanic stimulation [EGS] Electrotherapy utilizing direct current, or galvanism, resulting in muscle fiber contraction. Galvanism is also used for iontophoresis and the application of the current is used as a pain-relieving modality.

electromyography [EMG] The preparation or study of the graphic recording of the intrinsic electrical process that accompanies muscle contraction.

electrotherapy Use of electricity in treating disease: with direct current, galvanism; with alternating current, faradism.

elevator masticatory muscles Paired masseter, medial pterygoid, and temporalis muscles.

eminence [*syn:* **tubercle**] Prominence or projection of a bone.

emission scintigraphy Imaging process in which radiolabeled material is administered that is concentrated by the body in areas of rapid bone turnover.

endocrine Internal secretion from a gland directly into the systemic circulatory system.

endogenous Produced or originating from within a tissue or organism.

endoscope Instrument for examining the interior of a body cavity.

end-feel Quality of resistance felt in trajectory between full active opening and full passive opening, determined by gentle manipulation to increase range of motion (passive resistive stretch).

epidemiology Science concerned with defining and explaining the interrelationships of factors that determine disease frequency and distribution.

epilepsy Group of neurologic disorders characterized by recurrent episodes of convulsive seizures, sensory disturbance, abnormal behavior, and loss of consciousness.

equilibration of occlusion Adjustment of the dentition to evenly distribute the vertical and excursive forces of occlusion.

erosion of teeth Wearing away of dentition, especially by chemical means.

erythrocyte sedimentation rate [ESR] Rate at which red blood cells settle out in a tube of unclotted blood, expressed in millimeters per hour. Elevated sedimentation rate indicates the presence of inflammation, but is not specific for any disorder.

etiologic factors Factors that may be involved in, or cause, the development of a disease.

eustachian tube Opening from the middle ear cavity into the pharynx.

Ewing's sarcoma Malignant tumor that develops from bone marrow; most frequently in adolescent boys.

exacerbating factor Factor that increases the seriousness of a disease or disorder as marked by greater intensity in the signs or symptoms.

excursion of mandible Movement of the mandible away from the median or centric occlusion position.

lateral excursion Movement of the mandible to the side.

protrusive excursion Movement of the mandible forward.

extension of joint [*ant*: **flexion**] A motion that increases the joint angle.

external Away from the center of the body, outside a structure.

external auditory meatus Portion of the external ear contained within the head.

extracapsular [*ant*: **intracapsular**] Outside or external to the capsule.

extracranial Outside or external to the cranium.

extrinsic Originating outside of a part where it is found or on which it acts.

extrinsic trauma Trauma originating from outside an organ system or individual.

extrusion Process of forcing out of a normal position.

F

facebow Device used in dentistry for registering the relationship between the dentition and the facial skeleton, including the temporomandibular joint articulation, used to mount a dental cast on an articulator.

facet Small, smooth area on a hard surface.

facial Pertaining to the face or anterior part of the head from forehead to chin.

facial cranial nerve [CN VII] Mixed sensory and motor nerve that innervates the scalp, forehead, eyelids, muscles of facial expression, platysma muscle, submaxillary and submandibular salivary glands, and the afferent fibers from taste buds of the anterior two thirds of the tongue.

facial neuralgia [*unfavorable term*] See **atypical facial neuralgia**.

factitious disorder Sign, symptom, or disorder produced artificially; not natural.

fascia Collagenous connective tissue that encloses structures and separates them into various groups.

fasciculation Continuous muscle contraction.

fibrillation Involuntary recurrent contraction of individual muscle fibers.

fibrocartilage Type of cartilage in intervertebral discs, pubic symphysis, and mandibular symphysis, as well as on certain regions of the TMJ.

fibromyalgia [*syn*: **fibrositis, myofibrositis**] Nonarticular rheumatism with diffuse musculoskeletal aches and stiffness and exaggerated tenderness at multiple known anatomic sites, associated with nonrestorative sleep.

fibrosarcoma Sarcoma that contains connective tissue, develops suddenly from small nodules on the skin.

fibrosis Abnormal proliferation of fibrous connective tissue, occurs in the formation of scar tissue to replace normal tissue lost through injury or infection.

fibrositis [*syn*: **fibromyalgia myofibrositis**] See **fibromyalgia**.

fibrous Composed of or containing fibers of connective tissue.

fibrous dysplasia Abnormal fibrous replacement of osseous tissue with onset usually during childhood.

flexion [*ant*: **extension**] A motion that reduces the joint angle.

flexion-extension injury Traumatic, exaggerated movement of joints through extreme range of motion with hyperflexion and then hyperextension, resulting in ligamentous sprain, muscular strain, inflammation, and subsequent reflex muscle splinting.

fluoroscopy Radiographic technique for visualizing the contours and function of an organ or joint, providing immediate dynamic images.

fossa [*pl*, **fossae**] Hollow, pit, concavity, or depression, especially on the surface of the end of a bone.

freeway space Interocclusal distance or separation between the arches when the mandible is in its physiologic rest position.

fremitus Vibration.

frontal [*syn*: **coronal**] Vertical plane, perpendicular to sagittal plane, dividing the body into front to back portions.

G

genetic Pertaining to reproduction, birth, origin, or heredity.

geniculate neuralgia [*syn*: **nervous intermedius neuralgia, Ramsay Hunt's syndrome**] Painful disturbance of the sensory portion of the facial nerve characterized by lancinating pain deep to the ear.

giant cell arteritis [*syn*: **cranial arteritis**] Inflammation that fragments and distorts the arterial internal elastic lamina resulting in obliteration of the lumen. Not restricted to cranial arteries. Characterized by fever, anorexia, loss of weight, leucocytosis, and tenderness over the scalp and along facial and temporal arteries. May lead to blindness. Average age of onset is 70 years, uncommon before the age of 60 years, with 65% of reported cases in women.

ginglymoid Hinging joint with one convex and one concave surface, with movement in one plane of space.

gliding See **translation**.

glossodynia [*syn*: **glossalgia**] Painful or burning tongue.

glossopharyngeal neuralgia Severe, paroxysmal, lancinating pain of the branches of the glossopharyngeal nerve [CN IX] radiating to the throat, ear, teeth, and tongue. Rare, unilateral condition, usually in men over age of 50 years, that is triggered by movement in the tonsillar region by swallowing or coughing. Branches to the carotid artery can trigger vasovagal response including altered respiration, blood pressure, and cardiac output.

gnathic Pertaining to the jaw.

gnathologic Pertaining to the dynamics of the jaw.

gout Disorder of purine metabolism characterized by hyperuricemia and the deposition of monosodium urate crystals in joints, resulting in acute attacks of arthritis with red, hot, and swollen joints, especially the big toe. Occurs primarily in men over the age of 30 years.

grating joint sound See **crepitation**.

grinding of teeth [*syn*: **gritting**] See **attrition bruxism**.

H

hard tissue Skeletal tissue including bone, hyaline cartilage, and fibrocartilage.

headache See **cephalgia**.

hemarthrosis Bloody effusion into cavity of a joint.

hematoma A swelling or mass of blood confined to a tissue or space, caused by a break in a blood vessel.

hemifacial microsomia Condition in which one side of the face is abnormally small and underdeveloped, yet normally formed.

hemorrhage Abnormal internal or external discharge of blood.

herpes zoster Acute infection caused by the varicella zoster virus characterized by painful vesicular skin eruptions that follow the pathway of cranial or spinal nerves inflamed by the virus.

hinge axis Articulation about a single horizontal axis; for the mandible, a pure rotary movement on opening.

histaminic cephalgia See **cluster headache**.

history of present illness [HPI] Narrative report of each symptom or complaint including date of onset, duration, and character of the present illness.

homologous Corresponding or alike in critical attributes, similar in structure but not necessarily in function.

Horner's syndrome Neurologic condition characterized by unilateral miosis, ptosis, and facial anhydrosis, usually resulting from a cervical sympathetic lesion.

Horton's headache See **cluster headache**.

human leukocyte antigen-B27 [HLA-B27] Genetic marker usually present in individuals with ankylosing spondylitis.

humoral Relating to or arising from any of the body fluids.

hyaline cartilage Type of cartilage found on the articular surfaces of bones. Forms a template for endochondral bone formation.

hyperesthesia Increased sensitivity to sensory stimuli.

hyperextension Position of maximum or extreme extension of a joint.

hyperextension-hyperflexion injury Trauma that results in a combination of hyperextension and then hyperflexion of a joint and associated soft tissues.

hyperflexion Position of maximum or extreme flexion of a joint.

hyperfunction of muscle Increased function of muscle.

hypermobility [*ant*: **hypomobility**] Excessive mobility.

hypermobility syndrome Inherited arthropathy with traumatic synovitis associated with joint laxity; common in children but seldom persists into adult life.

hyperplasia Overdevelopment of tissue or structure with an increase in the number of normal cells.

hypertonicity of muscle Excess muscular tonus.

hypertrophy [*ant*: **atrophy**] Increase in size of an organ or structure that does not involve tumor formation. Increase in size or bulk is not from an increase in number of cells.

hyperuricemia Abnormal amount of uric acid in the blood, found in gout but also in many other conditions.

hypochondriasis Somatoform disorder marked by the preoccupation with and anxiety over one's health with exaggeration of normal sensations. Misinterpretation of normal physical signs and minor complaints as a serious illness or disease.

hypoglossal cranial nerve [CN XII] Mixed nerve carrying afferent proprioceptive impulses as well as efferent motor impulses to the intrinsic and extrinsic muscles of the tongue, with communication to the vagus nerve [CN X].

hypomobility [*ant*: **hypermobility**] Reduced or restricted mobility.

hypoplasia Incomplete or defective development or underdevelopment of a tissue or structure. Implies fewer than the usual number of cells.

hysterical trismus Severe restriction of mandibular motion due to acute psychologic distress.

I

iatrogenic Unfavorable response or condition caused by medical personnel, diagnostic tests, or treatment procedures.

idiopathic Pain, disease, or disorder of unknown origin or pathology.

idiopathic odontalgia Tooth pain without obvious pathology and of unknown etiology.

illness behavior Person experiencing symptoms seeks validation of and advice for treatment of the suspected disorder and adopts the sickness role.

imaging Representation or visual reproduction of a structure for purpose of diagnosis such as radiographs, ultrasound, CT, and MRI.

impairment Alteration of health status assessed by medical means.

incidence Number of new cases that occur during a specified period of time.

incisor The four front teeth of each arch, used for cutting.

infarct An area of tissue that undergoes necrosis following cessation of blood supply.

infection Invasion of a tissue by pathogenic microorganisms that reproduce and multiply, causing disease by local cellular injury, secretion of toxin, or antigen-antibody reaction in the host.

infectious arthritis Acute inflammatory condition of a joint caused by bacterial or viral infection.

inferior [*syn*: **caudal**, *ant*: **superior**] Tailward.

inflammation Protective response of tissue to irritation or injury that may be accompanied by redness, heat, swelling, and pain. Process initiates with increased vascular permeability with exudate of fluid from vessels.

initiating factors Factors that cause the onset of a disease or disorder.

insidious onset [*ant*: **acute onset**] Development that is gradual, subtle, or imperceptible.

insomnia Wakefulness, inability to sleep during the period when sleep should occur.

interarch Between two adjacent arches, as between the maxillary and mandibular dental arches.

intercuspal position [ICP] [*syn*: **centric occlusion**] Mandibular position with maximum interdigitation of opposing teeth.

interdisciplinary Multiple clinical specialties in one setting.

intermaxillary [*unfavorable term*] See **interocclusal**.

internal [*ant*: **external**] Toward the center of the body, within a structure.

internal derangement Localized mechanical fault interfering with smooth joint movement, including elongation, tear, or rupture of the capsule or ligaments causing altered disc position or morphology.

interocclusal Between the opposing dental arches.

interstitial Pertaining to the space between tissues.

intra-arch Located within an arch.

intra-articular Located within a joint.

intracapsular [*ant*: **extracapsular**] Located within the confines of the capsule of a joint.

intracranial [*ant*: **extracranial**] Within the cranium or skull.

intrameatal Within the auditory canal or meatus.

intraoral Within the oral cavity.

intrinsic [*ant*: **extrinsic**] Originating from or situated within an organ or tissue.

intrinsic trauma [*syn*: **microtrauma**, *ant*: **extrinsic trauma**] Trauma originating from within an organ system or individual.

ionizing radiation Radiation created by dislocating negatively charged electrons from atoms by the application of an electrical current.

iontophoresis Introduction of various ions into tissues through intact skin by means of direct electrical current.

ipsilateral [*syn*: **homolateral**, *ant*: **contralateral**] On the same side of the body.

isotonic exercises Active exercise without appreciable change in the force of muscle contraction, with shortening of the muscle.

isokinetic exercises Dynamic muscle activity performed at a constant angular velocity.

isometric exercises Active exercise performed against stable resistance, without change in the length of the muscle.

J

jaw Either or both bony structures, the maxilla or mandible, in which the teeth are set.

jaw tracking *[unfavorable term]* See **mandibular movement recording**.

juvenile rheumatoid arthritis [JRA] Represents 15% of cases of arthritis that begin before the age of 16 years, with rheumatoid factor found in 70% of cases. More common in women with onset most often between 12 to 15 years of age.

juxtaposed Positioned adjacently or side by side.

K

kinesiograph Instrument use to record and provide graphic representation of movement.

kinesiology The science or study of movement and the active and passive structures involved.

L

lacrimation Secretion of tears by the lacrimal glands.

larynx Air passageway connecting the pharynx with the trachea; the organ of voice.

latent disease Dormant disease; existing as a potential disease or disorder.

lateral *[ant: medial]* Away from the midline of the body.

lavage The process of washing out or irrigating a cavity.

leukocytosis Abnormal increase in the number of circulating white blood cells.

ligament Flexible band of fibrous tissue, slightly elastic and composed of parallel collagenous bundles, binding joints together and connecting various bones and cartilages.

locking of joint *[unfavorable term]* See **nonreducing disc**.

lupus erythematosus See **systemic lupus erythematosus**.

luxation Displacement of articular surfaces from normal position but with continued contact.

lysis Dissolution or loosening.

lytic Pertaining to lysis.

M

magnetic resonance imaging [MRI] Noninvasive, nonionizing imaging method that utilizes the signals from resonating hydrogen nuclei after they have been subjected to a charge in a magnetic field. Their relaxation and resultant resonant frequency is detected, measured, and converted by a computer into an image.

malformation Failure of proper or normal development, a primary structural defect that results from a localized error of morphogenesis.

malinger To feign an illness, usually to escape responsibility, provoke sympathy, or gain compensation.

malocclusion [See also **Angle's Classification**] Abnormal contact or position of the teeth of the maxillae with the teeth of the mandible.

mandible Horseshoe shaped lower jaw, consisting of the horizontal body joined at the symphysis and two vertical rami with the anterior coronoid process and the posterior condylar process, separated by the mandibular notch. The superior border of the body, the alveolus, contains sockets for the lower teeth.

mandibular movement recording Kinesiographic recording of the movement of the mandible.

mandibular orthopedic repositioning appliance [MORA] Interocclusal appliance, usually covering only the posterior mandibular teeth, that may be used to alter mandibular position.

mastication Process of chewing food in preparation for deglutition.

masticatory muscles Muscles responsible for masticatory motion including the paired masseter, temporalis, lateral pterygoid, and medial pterygoid muscles.

maxilla Upper jawbone, superior maxilla.

maxillofacial Pertaining to the maxilla and the face.

maxillomandibular Pertaining to the maxilla and mandible.

maximum intercuspation That position of the mandible relative to the maxillae where the greatest degree of tooth contact is achieved on articulation of the teeth.

medial [*ant*: **lateral**] Toward the midline of the body.

mediate auscultation Listening to sounds with the use of an instrument.

meniscectomy [*unfavorable term*] See **discectomy**.

mental disorder Disorder of mind or intellect, of psychologic or organic origin, that impairs adaptive functioning in area of emotional perception, cognitive behavior, or interpersonal relationships.

metaplasia Conversion of one tissue type into a form that is not normal for that tissue.

metastatic Shifting of a disease or its local manifestation from one part of the body to another. In cancer the appearance of neoplasms in parts of the body remote from the seat of the primary tumor.

micrognathia Abnormal smallness of the jaw, especially the lower jaw.

microtrauma [*syn*: **intrinsic trauma**] Minor trauma that may cause problems if repetitive, as distinguished from macrotrauma or gross trauma.

midline of teeth Interproximal contact zone between the central incisor teeth of the maxillary or mandibular dental arch.

migraine headache Paroxysmal, recurrent, intense headache, frequently unilateral and often accompanied by disordered vision and gastrointestinal disturbances. Headache variants classified by descriptive characteristics rather than by known physiologic mechanisms.

basilar migraine Disturbance of brain stem function with dramatic but slowly evolving neurologic events, often involving total blindness, altered consciousness, confusional states, and subsequent headache.

classic migraine with aura Headache with associated premonitory sensory, motor, or visual symptoms.

hemiplegic migraine Oculomotor nerve palsy and partial to complete paralysis of motor function.

ophthalmoplegic migraine Nonthrobbing orbital or periorbital pain that radiates to the hemicranium, often accompanied by vomiting, lasting 1 to 4 days. Frequently accompanied by ipsilateral ptosis and sometimes by pupillary dilatation.

retinal migraine Repeated attacks of monocular scotoma or blindness lasting less than 1 hour.

common migraine without aura Condition in which no focal neurologic disturbance precedes the headache.

mixed connective tissue disease See **connective tissue disorder**.

mobilization of a joint Restoration of motion to a joint.

monosynaptic reflex Simplest and fastest reflex involving one motor and one sensory neuron with one synapse, eg, muscle stretch reflex.

mood disturbance Disturbance of the emotional state of an individual.

morphology Form or structure of an organism.

motor neuron A neuron carrying impulses that initiate muscle contraction.

multidisciplinary Different specialties in multiple clinical settings.

multifactorial Resulting from the combined action of several factors.

multiple myeloma Malignant neoplasm of bone marrow.

multiple sclerosis Chronic, slowly progressive disease of the central nervous system of unknown etiology, characterized by demyelinated glial patches called plaques.

muscle Tissue comprised of contractile fibers that effect movements of an organ or part of the body. Muscle types include striated skeletal and cardiac muscles and smooth, nonstriated visceral muscles.

digastric muscle Origin at the digastric notch of the mastoid process with insertion on the mandible near the symphysis, raises the hyoid bone and base of the tongue and depresses the mandible.

lateral (external) pterygoid muscle Origin at the lateral pterygoid plate and greater wing of the sphenoid with insertion at the fovea of the condyle and capsule of the temporomandibular joint. Muscle of mastication that translates the mandible and is active on mouth opening and near final mouth closure.

masseter muscle Origin of the superficial masseter on the zygomatic process and arch with insertion on the ramus and the angle of the lower jaw. Origin of the deep masseter on the zygomatic arch with insertion on the upper half of the ramus and the coronoid process of the lower jaw. Powerful muscle of mastication that elevates the mandible.

medial pterygoid muscle Origin on the maxillary tuberosity and medial surface of the lateral pterygoid plate with insertion on the medial surface of the ramus and angle of the mandible. Muscle of mastication that elevates and protrudes the mandible and is active in mandibular movements during speech.

scalene muscles Origin on the transverse process of the cervical vertebrae with insertion on the ribs. Acts to stabilize the cervical vertebra or incline the neck to the side.

sternocleidomastoid muscle Rotates and extends the head and flexes the vertebral column. Origin on the sternum and clavicle with insertion on the mastoid process and superior nuchal line of the occipital bone.

suboccipital muscles Muscles situated below the occipital bone that act to stabilize the cervical vertebrae and head position.

suprahyoid muscles Digastric, geniohyoid, mylohyoid, and stylohyoid, all attach to the upper part of the hyoid bone and act to stabilize and elevate the hyoid bone and depress the mandible.

temporal muscle Origin on the temporal fossa with the insertion on the coronoid process and anterior aspect of the ramus. Muscle of mastication that elevates and retrudes the mandible.

trapezius muscle Origin on the superior nuchal line of the occipital bone, spinous process of the seventh cervical and all the thoracic vertebrae with insertion on the clavicle and scapula. Elevates the shoulder and rotates the scapula.

muscle cramp [*unfavorable term*] See **myospasm**.

muscular dystrophy Group of genetically transmitted diseases characterized by progressive atrophy of symmetric groups of skeletal muscles without evidence of degeneration of neural tissue.

musculoskeletal Relating to the muscles and skeleton.

myalgia Pain in a muscle.

myelin Fatty substance that forms a major component of the sheath that surrounds and insulates the axon of some nerve cells.

myoclonus Clonic spasm or twitching that results from the contraction of one or more muscle groups.

myofascial Pertaining to muscle and its attaching fascia.

myofascitis Inflammation of muscle and its fascia.

myofibrositis See **fibromyalgia**.

myogenous Having origin in muscle.

miosis Contraction of the sphincter of the iris, causing the pupil to constrict.

myositis Inflammation of muscle tissue.

myositis ossificans Ossification of a hematoma, usually after injury, located in but not involving muscle.

myospasm [*syn*: **acute trismus, muscle cramp**] Spasmodic contraction of a muscle.

myxoma Neoplasm derived from connective tissue, composed of a mucoid matrix.

N

natural history of disorder The natural sequence, duration, transitional stages, and nature of change of a disease or disorder over time, without external interference such as trauma or treatment.

neoplasm [*syn:* **tumor**] Abnormal growth of new tissue, benign or malignant.

nervous intermedius neuralgia [*syn:* **geniculate neuralgia, Ramsay Hunt's syndrome**] See **geniculate neuralgia**.

neuralgia [*syn:* **neurodynia**] Pain of severe throbbing or stabbing character in the distribution of a nerve.

neuritis Inflammation of a nerve that may cause neuralgia, hyperesthesia, anesthesia, paralysis, muscular atrophy, and impaired reflexes.

neurolepsis Altered state of consciousness, as induced by a neuroleptic medication, characterized by quiescence, reduced motor activity, anxiety, and indifference to the surroundings.

neurologic Pertaining to the nervous system and its disorders.

neurolysis Destruction of nerve tissue or loosening of adhesions surrounding a nerve.

neuromuscular Concerning both nerves and muscles.

neuropathy Disease of the nerves characterized by inflammation and degeneration of the peripheral nerves.

neuropathic pain Pain resulting from a neurologic disorder or disease.

neurovascular Concerning both the nervous and vascular systems.

nightguard appliance Interocclusal appliance traditionally worn only at night to reduce adverse effects of bruxism.

nociceptive Capable of receiving and transmitting painful sensation.

nocturnal [*ant:* **diurnal**] Pertaining to or occurring in the hours of darkness.

noninnervated Tissue that is lacking in a sensory or motor nerve supply.

noninvasive Denoting diagnostic or therapeutic procedures that do not require penetrating the skin or entering a cavity or organ of the body.

nonsteroidal anti-inflammatory drug [**NSAID**] Class of anti-inflammatory medications that also provide analgesia, useful in the treatment of musculoskeletal disorders.

nonworking occlusal contact Tooth contact on the contralateral side during guided lateral excursive movement of the mandible.

nuchal line Bony ridge at the nape or back of the skull.

O

occipital neuralgia Neuralgia of the greater occipital nerve, a continuation of the dorsal ramus of the second cervical nerve that emerges onto the scalp between the sternocleidomastoid and trapezius muscles, midway between the occipital protuberance and the mastoid process.

occlusal adjustment Equilibration or grinding of the occluding surfaces of teeth.

occlusal appliance See **interocclusal appliance**.

occlusal guidance Tooth-determined guidance of the mandible in eccentric movements, when the teeth remain in contact.

occlusal vertical dimension [**OVD**] The vertical position of the mandible relative to the maxilla and facial skeleton when the teeth are interdigitated.

occlusion Alignment of the mandibular and maxillary teeth when the jaw is closed or in functional contact.

ocular Pertaining to the eye.

odontogenic Derived from or produced in the teeth or tissues that produce the teeth.

open bite Abnormal dental condition in which the anterior teeth do not contact when the posterior teeth are brought into occlusion.

opthalmic Pertaining to the eye.

oral Pertaining to the mouth.

organic Related to the organs of the body.

orofacial Relating to the mouth and face.

orthodontic Pertaining to the prevention of and correction of irregularities and malocclusion of the teeth.

orthognathic Pertaining to malposition of the bones of the jaws.

orthopedic Relating to form and function of the locomotor structures, especially the extremities, spine, and associated structures including bones, joints, muscles, fascia, ligaments, and cartilage.

orthopedic appliance See **orthotic**.

orthostatic Relating to an erect or upright position.

orthotic Mechanical appliance or splint for orthopedic use to support or improve the function of part of the body.

osseous Bony.

ossification Development of bone.

osteoarthritis A chronic disease resulting in joint deformity caused by disintegration and abrasion of articular cartilage. In late stage is accompanied by proliferation of new skeletal tissue at the margins of the joint surface, known as marginal osteophytes, lipping, or spurs. Not a disorder of cartilage, but the consequences of repetitive microfractures sustained by bone during high-impact loading. The cartilage fibrillation and breakdown is not an inflammatory process, but the breakdown is accompanied by inflammation.

osteoarthrosis Noninflammatory joint disorder characterized by progressive deterioration and loss of articular cartilage and subchondral bone, may be accompanied by proliferation of new bone and soft tissue.

osteoblast Bone-forming cell derived from mesenchyme.

osteoblastoma Benign, vascularized tumor of poorly formed bone and fibrous tissue that causes resorption of native bone.

osteoclast Multinucleated cell that causes absorption and removal of bone.

osteoma A benign slow-growing mass of mature bone, usually arising from the skull or mandible.

osteomyelitis Inflammation of bone, especially of the marrow, caused by pathogenic organisms.

osteophyte Marginal adaptation of joint formed by new skeletal tissue.

osteosarcoma A malignant bone tumor comprised of anaplastic cells derived from mesenchyme.

osteotomy Incision or cutting through a bone.

otolaryngology Division of medical science concerned with diseases of the ear, larynx, upper respiratory tract, and other head and neck structures.

otologic Pertaining to the ear.

overbite Vertical overlap of anterior teeth.

overjet Horizontal overlap of anterior teeth.

P

Paget's disease Disorder of unknown etiology with inflammation of one or many bones, resulting in thickening and softening of bones with unorganized bone repair.

pain Unpleasant sensory and emotional experience triggered by noxious stimulation of sensory nerve endings, usually from tissue damage.

pain mediator factors Neurovascular substances activated by noxious stimuli that trigger or sustain pain. Include leukotriene B4 [LTB4], prostaglandin E2 [PCE2], platelet-activating Factor[PAF], and substance P.

palliative Mitigating, reducing the severity of, or denoting the elimination of symptoms without curing the underlying disease.

palpation Examination by feeling with the hands; perceiving by the sense of touch.

palsy Paralysis, often connoting paresis.

panic disorder [*syn*: **anxiety disorder**] Violent and unreasoning anxiety and fear, with the person unable to organize any defense or coping skills.

panoramic radiograph Circular tomography that images the jaws and related structures.

pantograph Dental device that incorporates a pair of facebows fixed to the jaws, used for recording mandibular movement patterns and centric jaw relationships.

parafunction Nonfunctional activity including clenching and grinding (bruxism) or rhythmic chewing-like empty mouth movements.

paralysis Palsy, loss of power or voluntary movement in muscle through injury or disease of its nerve supply.

paravertebral Alongside or near the vertebral column.

paresis Partial or incomplete paralysis.

paresthesia Altered sensation, such as burning, prickling, tickling, or tingling.

parotid gland Paired salivary gland located superficial to the masseter and extending from in front of the ear to down below the angle of the mandible.

paroxysmal Sudden onset of a symptom or disease, with recurrent manifestations. A sharp jabbing pain, spasm, or convulsion.

passive range of motion Motion imparted to an articulation, an associated capsule, ligaments, and muscles by another individual, machine, or outside force.

passive resistive stretch Activity designed to increase muscle strength by activating the muscle against an opposing force.

pathognomonic Special characteristic or symptom of a disease.

pathophysiologic derangement of function Alteration of function seen in disease as distinguished from structural alteration.

pathologic Diseased, morbid, causing disease or pathosis.

pathosis Diseased state or condition.

periarticular Surrounding a joint.

pericranium Fibrous membrane surrounding the cranium, periosteum of the skull.

periodontium The connective tissue between a tooth and the alveolar bone.

peripheral nervous system The motor and sensory nerves and ganglia outside the brain and spinal cord, consisting of 12 pairs of cranial nerves, 31 pairs of spinal nerves, and their various branches in body organs.

perpetuating factors Factors that interfere with resolution of or enhance the progression of a disease or disorder.

pharmacotherapy Treatment of disease or disorder by means of drugs.

pharynx Passageway for air from the nasal cavity to the larynx.

phonophobia Abnormal sensitiveness to sound.

photophobia Abnormal sensitiveness to light, especially of the eyes.

physical therapy [*syn*: **physiotherapy**] Treatment with physical and mechanical means such as massage, manipulation, exercise, heat, cold, ultrasound, and electricity.

Pierre Robin syndrome Unusual smallness of the jaw combined with cleft palate, downward displacement of the tongue, and an absent gag reflex, characterized by respiratory obstruction in infants.

pinna [*syn*: **auricle**] External ear.

placebo effect Physical or emotional change occurring after a substance is taken or a treatment is provided, with the change not directly attributable to any specific property of the substance or effect of the therapeutic agent.

planar scintigraphy Imaging process in which area of interest is scanned with a gamma camera 2 to 4 hours after the administration of a radioactive material.

platelet aggravating factor [**PAF**] Produced by reaction of antigen on IgE-sensitized basophiles, which aggregates platelets and is a factor in producing inflammation.

plication The stitching of folds or tucks in a tissue to reduce its size, as in the retrodiscal tissue of the temporomandibular joint, in an attempt to reposition a displaced articular disc.

polyarthritis Inflammation of more than one joint.

polymyalgia rheumatica Pain and stiffness of the proximal limbs that evolves insidiously over weeks or months or acute onset with myalgia and fever. Onset may be unilateral but invariably becomes bilateral. Successive involvement of muscle groups with morning stiffness. Muscle strength is unimpaired and electromyographic findings and serum enzyme levels are normal.

polysynaptic reflex Neural conduction pathway formed by a chain of many synaptically connected nerve cells.

posterior ligament [*unfavorable term*] See **retrodiscal tissue**.

postherpetic neuralgia Neuralgia caused by persistent varicella zoster virus that remains latent in nerve ganglia until the host's immunity has waned.

postsurgical neuralgia [*syn*: **anesthesia do-**

lorosa] Loss of sensation of a part but with paradoxical pain following surgical intervention.

posterior [*ant*: **anterior**] Relating to the back or dorsal side of the human body.

preauricular Located in front of the auricle of the ear.

predisposing Indicating a tendency or susceptibility to develop a certain condition in the presence of specific environmental stimuli.

predisposing factors Factors that increase the risk of developing a disease or disorder.

prevalence Number of cases of a disease or disorder at a given point in time, usually measured as a ratio of the positive cases to the number of people in the population of interest at that point in time.

prodrome Early or premonitory symptom indicative of an approaching event or disorder.

prognathic Having a forward projecting jaw or jaws relative to the craniofacial skeleton.

prostaglandins Fatty acids that are extremely active biologic substances with effects on the cardiovascular, gastrointestinal, respiratory, and central nervous system.

prosthetic Pertaining to the replacement of a missing part or augmentation of a deficient part by an artificial substitute.

protective splinting of muscle [*syn*: **reflex splinting**] A reflexive contraction of adjacent muscles to prevent movement or stabilize the tissue, resulting from noxious stimuli of a sensory field of a joint, soft tissue, or other structure.

proteoglycan Mucopolysaccharides bound to protein chains in covalent complexes occurring in the extracellular matrix of connective tissue.

protrusion State of being thrust forward or projected, moving the mandible forward of centric position.

provocation test Diagnostic method of inducing an episode or aggravating a symptom by provoking a tissue or system.

proximal [*ant*: **distal**] Close to or toward the origin.

pseudoankylosis [*syn*: **fibrous ankylosis**] See **ankylosis**.

pseudogout Condition in which calcified deposits in synovial fluid, articular cartilage, and adjacent soft tissues, free from urate and consisting of calcium hypophosphate crystals, leads to gout-like attacks of pain and swelling of the involved joints.

psoriatic arthritis Polyarticular, progressive erosive joint inflammation with associated psoriatic skin lesions.

psychic trauma Emotional shock, injury, or stressful situation that produces a lasting impression, especially on the subconscious mind.

psychogenic pain disorders Characterized by persistent and severe pain for which there is no apparent physical cause. May be accompanied by sensory or motor dysfunction.

psychosocial Involving both psychological and social aspects of functioning in society.

psychotic Affected by psychosis or mental disorder causing gross distortion or disorganization of a person's mental capacity, affective response, and capacity to recognize reality and to communicate with others. Difficulty coping with the everyday demands of life.

psychotropic medications Drugs affecting the mind, used to treat mental disorders.

ptosis Prolapse or drooping of upper eyelid from altered third cranial nerve function or cervical portion of the autonomic nervous system.

pulpitis Inflammation of the tooth pulp tissue.

R

radionuclides Atoms that disintegrate by emission of electromagnetic radiation, used in radiographic studies.

radiograph See **roentgenogram**.

Ramsay Hunt's syndrome [*syn*: **nervous intermedius neuralgia, geniculate neuralgia**] See **geniculate neuralgia**.

range of motion [**ROM**] The range, measured in degrees of a circle, through which a joint can be extended of flexed. Commonly reported in millimeters rather than in degrees with reference to the TMJ.

rapid eye movement [REM] sleep Active stage of sleep, characterized by prominent increase in the variability of heart rate, respiration, and blood pressure, all of which are very regular and at low levels in non-REM sleep. Phasic REM sleep includes periods of rapid eye movements and muscle twitching.

reciprocal clicking Clicking noise during mandibular opening and again during closing, usually just before the teeth occlude.

recruitment of muscle Greater or sustained muscle activity in response to prolonged or increased stimulus to a given receptor or afferent nerve causing increase in the number and size of active motor units of a given muscle.

reducing disc [*ant*: **nonreducing disc**] Temporary repositioning of the articular disc of the TMJ, approximating its normal functional relationship to the condyle during mandibular movements.

referred pain Heterotropic pain, felt in an area other than the site of origin.

reflex splinting of muscle [*syn*: **protective splinting**] Restricted or guarded joint movement due to reflex rigidity of muscles as a means of avoiding pain caused by movement.

reflex sympathetic dystrophy [RSD] Specific group of painful disorders precipitated by an injury to peripheral tissues and sustained by neural mechanisms. Characterized by progressive autonomic dysfunction including changes in cutaneous temperature, color, texture, and perspiration followed by trophic changes in the skin, muscle, and bone.

Reiter's syndrome Triad of arthritis, urethritis, and conjunctivitis that usually follows nonspecific urethritis. Polyarticular and occurs predominately in men.

relaxed position of mandible See **rest position**.

remodeling Adaptive alteration of tissue form secondary to functional demands through cellular response of articular cartilage and subchondral bone.

repositioning appliance Interocclusal appliance that alters mandibular position.

rest position of mandible [*syn*: **relaxed position, physiologic rest position**] Postural relation of the mandible to the maxilla when the patient is resting comfortably in an upright position, with the condyles in a neutral, unstrained position in the glenoid fossa and the mandibular musculature in a state of minimum tonic contraction to maintain the posture.

restorative Pertaining to the repair, reconstruction, or replacement of the dentition.

retrodiscal tissue [*syn*: **bilaminar zone**] Loose connective tissue rich in interstitial collagen fibers, adipose tissue, arteries, and a venous plexus. Attaches to the posterior band of the articular disc, extending to the posterior capsule of the TMJ, consisting of an elastic superior lamina and a ligamentous inferior lamina.

retrognathia Facial disharmony in which one or both jaws, usually the mandible, are posterior to normal in their craniofacial relationship.

retruded contact position [RCP] [*syn*: **centric relation, centric relation occlusion**] Point of initial tooth contact when the mandible is guided into a hinged or retruded position on closure.

review of systems [ROS] A system-by-system review of body functions while completing the health history and physical examination.

rheumatoid arthritis Chronic polyarticular erosive disease characterized by bilateral involvement with proliferative synovitis, more common in women.

rheumatoid factor [RhF] Antigamma globulin antibodies found in the serum of most patients with rheumatoid arthritis but also occurs in a small percentage of apparently normal individuals and with other collagen vascular diseases, chronic infections, and noninfectious diseases.

risk factor Factor that causes an individual or a group to be vulnerable to a disease or disorder, increasing the incidence or severity of the event.

roentgenogram [*syn*: **radiograph**] Image produced by x-rays striking a sensitized film after passing through a structure.

rostral [*syn*: **superior, cephalic**, *ant*: **caudal**] Toward the head.

rotation To move about an axis.

rotation of condyle Part of mandibular opening path, starting at maximum intercuspation, prior to translation or protrusive movement of the condyle. Can occur before, during, or after condylar translation. Full mandibular ROM requires a combination of rotation and translation. Rotation occurs primarily between condyle and the inferior surface of disc.

S

sagittal Anteroposterior direction.

sarcoidosis Chronic infectious disease of unknown cause marked by granulomatous lesions in the skin, lymph nodes, salivary glands, eyes, lungs, and bones.

scintigraphy Process in which image is derived from measuring a radioactive isotope, revealing its concentration in a specific organ or tissue.

scintillation detector Device for measuring radioactivity that relies on the emission of light or ultraviolet radiation from a crystal subjected to ionizing radiation.

scleroderma Skin disease in which thickened, hard, rigid, and pigmented patches occur due to an increase in the connective tissue of the corium and subcutaneous structures.

scotoma Isolated area of varying size and shape, within the visual field, in which vision is absent or depressed.

secondary gain Indirect benefit, usually obtained through an illness or debility, that may include monetary and disability benefits, personal attentions, or escape from unpleasant situations and responsibilities.

sedimentation rate See **erythrocyte sedimentation rate**.

sensory nerve Afferent fibers that conduct sensory impulses from the periphery of the body to the brain or spinal cord.

serology Study of blood serum or exudate.

shingles [*unfavorable term*] See **postherpetic neuralgia**.

sialography Radiographic technique in which a salivary gland is filmed after an opaque substance is injected into its duct.

signs An objective clinical finding as perceived by an examiner.

single photon emission computed tomography [SPECT] Similar to a CT scan except that the radiation source is inside the area of interest rather than external.

sinusitis Inflammation of the mucosa of the paranasal sinuses.

Sjögren's syndrome Collagen disorder that is characterized by atrophic changes of the lacrimal and salivary glands, resulting in dryness of the eyes and xerostomia, more common in women and sometimes with associated rheumatoid arthritis.

skeletal Pertaining to bone, cartilage, and supporting soft tissue.

sleep apnea Breathing abnormality occurring during sleep, commonly related to upper airway obstruction but may be related to central apnea, characterized by cessation of airflow secondary to a lack of respiratory effort.

soft tissue Skeletal tissue including muscles and their fascial envelopes, tendons, tendon sheaths, ligaments, joint capsule, and bursae.

somatic Pertaining to the body as distinct from the mind or psyche. Pertaining to the structures of the body wall, eg, skeletal tissue in contrast to visceral structures.

somatization Process of expressing a disturbed mental condition as a disturbed bodily function.

somatoform disorders Conditions in which psychogenic symptoms resemble those of physical disease. The physical symptoms suggest the presence of a physical disorder but there are no organic findings. The symptoms are not under voluntary control, unlike the symptoms occurring in factitious disorders. The DSM-IIIR recognizes five disorders in this group: body dysmorphic disorder, conversion disorder, hypochondriasis, somatization disorder, somatoform pain disorder.

somatopsychic Pertaining to both body and mind, denoting a physical disorder that produces mental symptoms.

sonography Recording of sound through the use of ultrasonography.

space occupying lesion Abnormal mass or

tumor that distends adjacent tissue as it enlarges.

spasm of muscle Involuntary, sudden movement or convulsive muscle contraction. Spasm may be clonic (characterized by alternating contraction and relaxation), tonic (sustained), or tetanic (prolonged, sustained involuntary contraction without interruption).

sphenoid bone Compound, unpaired wedge-shaped bone at the base of the cranium separating the frontal and ethmoid bones and maxillas frontally from the temporal and occipital bones at the back.

spinal accessory cranial nerve [CN 11] Motor nerve comprised of cranial and spinal branches that supply the trapezius, sternomastoid muscles, and pharynx.

splint [*syn*: **orthosis**] Rigid or flexible appliance or device to immobilize, support, protect, or correct injured, displaced, or deformed structures.

splinting of muscle Reducing motion of the painful part as protection against pain.

spondylarthropathy Disease of the joints of the spine or intervertebral articulations.

spontaneous remission Resolution of signs or symptoms of disease occurring unaided, without treatment.

spray and stretch Physical therapy technique utilizing vapocoolant spray followed by passive muscle stretch.

stabilization appliance Intraoral appliance utilized to control joint or muscle symptoms during period of time required for mandibular position or a temporomandibular joint disorder to stabilize.

standard of care Established model or guidelines that identify the process and anticipated outcome of care in a given community or setting.

stellate ganglion Star shaped ganglion located between the transverse process of the seventh cervical vertebra and the head of the first rib with postganglionic fibers running to the carotid, middle ear, salivary and lacrimal glands, and the ciliary ganglion via cranial nerves IX, X, and XI, and the upper three cervical nerves.

Still's disease Seronegative arthritis, often accompanied by fever and rash, representing 70% of cases of arthritis that begin before the age of 16 years.

stomatognathic Denoting the mouth and jaws collectively.

stress Sum of the biologic reactions to any adverse stimulus—physical, mental, emotional, internal, or external—that tend to disturb the homeostasis of an organism. When the reactions are inappropriate, they may lead to disease states.

stressor Cause of stress, any factor that disturbs homeostasis.

subcondylar osteotomy [*syn*: **condylotomy**] Surgical section beneath or below the condylar head.

subluxation Partial or incomplete dislocation in which the joint surfaces remain in partial contact. Relaxation or stretching of the capsule and ligaments of the temporomandibular joint that results in popping noise during movement.

submandibular Situated below the mandible.

superior [*syn*: **rostral**, *ant*: **inferior**] Situated above or upward, nearer the vertex.

superior laryngeal neuralgia Condition characterized by paroxysmal, unilateral submandibular pain that may radiate to the ear, eye or shoulder, a distribution indistinguishable from glossopharyngeal neuralgia. The superior laryngeal nerve is a branch of the vagus nerve [CN X] and innervates the cricothyroid muscle of the larynx.

symmetry Correspondence in size, shape, and relative position on opposite sides of the body.

sympathectomy [*syn*: **neurolysis**] Excision or interruption of some portion of the sympathetic nervous pathway.

sympathetic nervous system Division of the autonomic nervous system originating in the thoracic and first few lumbar spinal cord segments. System prepares for "fight or flight" reaction to stress.

symptoms Indication of a disease as perceived by a patient. A subjective symptom is one perceptible only to the patient, such as vertigo. An objective symptom is perceptible to patient and others.

synapse Junction between the processes of two neurons or a neuron and an effector organ.

syndrome Grouping of symptoms or signs of disorder function relating to one another by means of some anatomic, physiologic, or biochemical peculiarity. Combination of symptoms resulting from a single cause.

synostosis [*syn:* **bony ankylosis**] Normal or abnormal fusion of adjacent bones by osseous material.

synovial Containing a clear, thick lubricating fluid in a joint, bursa, or tendon sheath secreted by the membrane lining the cavity or sheath.

synovial chondromatosis Rare condition in which cartilage nodules develop in the connective tissue below the synovial membranes. The cartilage foci on the surface of the synovium may detach and result in loose bodies within the joint.

synovial fluid Produced by the synovium to bathe the tendons, articular surfaces, and attachment tissue to provide nutrition and reduce friction.

synovial osteochondromatosis See **synovial chondromatosis**.

synovitis Inflammation of the synovial lining related to infection. Immunologic condition or secondary to cartilage degeneration or trauma.

synovium Synovial membrane.

systemic disease Disease affecting the entire organism as distinguished from any of its individual parts.

systemic lupus erythematosus [**SLE**] Chronic inflammatory condition affecting many organ systems, including lesions of the skin, vasculitis, and renal and neurologic involvement.

T

tardive dyskinesia Involuntary, repetitious movements of the muscles of the face, the limbs, and the trunk, most often related to the use of phenothiazine medications.

temporal Pertaining to the temples.

temporal arteritis [*unfavorable term*] See **giant cell arteritis, cranial arteritis**.

temporal bone Paired, large bone forming the lower part of the cranium and consisting of four portions—the mastoid, the squama, the petrous, and the tympanic.

temporomandibular [**TM**] See **temporomandibular joint**.

temporomandibular disorder [**TMD**] Collective term embracing a number of clinical problems that involve the masticatory muscles, the temporomandibular joint, or both. Common patient complaints include jawache, headache, earache, and face pain and there may be associated limited or asymmetric jaw movement and joint sounds.

temporomandibular joint [**TMJ**] Paired joint, articulating the mandibular condyle, articular disc, and squamous portion of the temporal bone, capable of gliding and hinge movements.

tendomyositis Inflammatory condition of a tendon and its associated muscle.

tendon Strong, flexible, and inelastic fibrous band of tissue attaching muscle to bone.

tendinitis Inflammatory condition of a tendon, usually resulting from strain.

tension-type headache Head pain devoid of migrainous characteristics. Usually bilateral and historically associated with muscle tension and occurring in relationship to emotional conflict.

thermography Graphic representation of the skin temperature variations between adjacent tissues or between the same area on two sides of the body.

tic douloureux See **trigeminal neuralgia**.

time-contingent basis Prescription of medication or other treatment on a regular, time-related basis, rather than on the patient's perceived need for medication or treatment because of pain severity.

tinnitus Subjective ringing, buzzing, or roaring sound in the ear.

tomography Radiographic technique for representing a detailed cross section at a predetermined depth and thickness of cut. Accomplished by moving the film and the x-ray source in opposite directions during the exposure, blurring the structures in front of and behind the area of interest.

Towne's radiograph Fronto-occipital plain film projection of the skull.

transcranial radiograph Plain film projection of the contralateral mandibular condyle from a superior angulation.

transcutaneous electrical nerve stimulation translation [TENS] Low voltage stimulation used as therapy.

translation of condyle [*syn*: **gliding**] Mandibular movement associated with protrusive or forward movement of the condyle. Can occur before, during, or after condylar rotation. Protrusion or lateral excursion can consists of pure translation with no rotation of mandible. In normal TMJ the movement occurs primarily between the superior aspect of the disc and the articular tubercle.

traumatic arthritis Arthritis that is the direct result of an injury, affecting normal joints or aggravating existing joint disease or derangement.

Treacher-Collins syndrome Inherited disorder characterized by mandibular and facial dysostosis.

trigeminal cranial nerve [CN V] Somatosensory innervation for structures embryologically derived from the first brachial arch including the oral cavity and the face. Innervation by three main branches—the opthalmic (V_1), maxillary (V_2), and mandibular (V_3) branches. The motor fibers of this mixed nerve principally supply the muscles of mastication as well as the mylohyoid, anterior belly of the digastric, the tensor veli palatini, and the tenor tympani muscles.

trigeminal neuralgia [*syn*: **tic douloureux**] Disorder of the sensory divisions of the trigeminal nerve, characterized by recurrent paroxysms of sharp, stabbing pains in the distribution of one or more branches of the nerve.

trigger point Irritable focus in a soft tissue structure, most commonly muscle, that when stimulated elicits referred pain.

trismus Limited mouth opening resulting from tonic contraction of the muscles of mastication that may occur with infection, encephalitis, inflammation of salivary glands, or tetanus.

trophic Pertaining to nutrition or nourishment of a tissue.

tubercle [*syn*: **eminence**] Small rounded elevation on a bone.

tumor See **neoplasm**.

U

ultrasonography Delineation of structures by measurement of the reflection or transmission of high frequency ultrasonic waves at interfaces between adjacent structures.

ultrasound Sound waves of frequency higher than the range audible to the human ear or above 20,000 vibrations per second (Hz).

unilateral [*ant*: **bilateral**] Occurring on one side only.

urate crystals Salt of uric acid that may be deposited in gouty joints.

V

vagus cranial nerve [CN X] Afferent and efferent mixed nerve that exits via the jugular foramen and sends parasympathetic branches to the viscera as well as the muscles of the pharynx and larynx.

vapocoolant spray Spray that acts as a counterirritant because of the extreme coldness of the solution on evaporation when applied over the skin.

vascular Pertaining to a blood vessel.

vasculitis Inflammatory condition of a blood vessel.

vertical dimension of occlusion [VDO] The vertical height or position of the mandible with the teeth in occlusion as measured relative to the facial skeleton.

vertigo Sensation of irregular or whirling

motions, either of oneself or of external objects, disturbance of equilibrium.

W

whiplash [*unfavorable term*] See **flexion-extension injury**.

working occlusal contact Tooth contact on the ipsilateral side during guided lateral excursive movement of the mandible.

X

xerostomia Dryness of the mouth.

Z

zygoma Area formed by the union of the zygomatic bone and the zygomatic process of the temporal bone and the maxillary bone.